Chapter 1: Introduction to Oncology

Overview of Cancer Biology and the Importance of Treatment Modalities

Cancer remains one of the most formidable health challenges globally, affecting millions of people and their families each year. Understanding the underlying biology of cancer is crucial for mastering effective treatment strategies, including radiotherapy and chemotherapy. This chapter provides an overview of cancer biology, the complexity of the disease, and the critical role that various treatment modalities play in managing cancer effectively.

The Nature of Cancer

At its core, cancer is characterized by uncontrolled cell growth and division. Normal cells undergo a regulated cycle of growth, division, and death. In contrast, cancer cells evade these controls, leading to the formation of tumors. These tumors can be benign (non-cancerous) or malignant (cancerous), with malignant tumors having the potential to invade surrounding tissues and metastasize to distant sites in the body.

The transformation of a normal cell into a cancerous one involves multiple genetic mutations, often triggered by a combination of genetic predisposition and environmental factors, such as exposure to carcinogens (cancer-causing agents), lifestyle choices (e.g., smoking, diet), and infectious agents (e.g., certain viruses). These mutations affect key regulatory pathways that govern cell proliferation, differentiation, and apoptosis (programmed cell death), resulting in the hallmark features of cancer, including:

1. **Sustained proliferative signaling**: Cancer cells can continually signal themselves or neighboring cells to divide and grow.
2. **Evading growth suppressors**: Cancer cells can ignore signals that normally halt cell growth and division.
3. **Resisting cell death**: Cancer cells develop mechanisms to evade apoptosis, allowing them to survive longer than normal cells.
4. **Enabling replicative immortality**: Cancer cells can divide indefinitely, unlike normal cells that have a limited lifespan.
5. **Inducing angiogenesis**: Cancer cells can promote the formation of new blood vessels to supply nutrients and oxygen to growing tumors.
6. **Activating invasion and metastasis**: Cancer cells can invade neighboring tissues and spread to other parts of the body, complicating treatment efforts.

The Importance of Treatment Modalities

Given the complexity of cancer biology, effective treatment often requires a multidisciplinary approach. The primary goals of cancer treatment are to eliminate cancer cells, prevent their spread, and manage symptoms to enhance the patient's quality of life. The main treatment modalities include:

1. **Surgery**: The surgical removal of tumors is often the first line of treatment for localized cancers. It can provide immediate relief from symptoms and is curative in certain cases.
2. **Radiotherapy**: This modality uses high-energy radiation to target and kill cancer cells. It can be used as a primary treatment, adjuvant therapy after surgery, or palliative care to alleviate symptoms in advanced cases.
3. **Chemotherapy**: Involving the use of cytotoxic drugs, chemotherapy aims to kill rapidly dividing cancer cells. It can be administered alone or in combination with other therapies to improve outcomes.
4. **Targeted Therapy**: This approach utilizes drugs that specifically target cancer cell mechanisms or markers, leading to more effective treatment with fewer side effects.
5. **Immunotherapy**: Harnessing the body's immune system, immunotherapy enhances the ability to recognize and attack cancer cells, representing a significant advancement in oncology.
6. **Palliative Care**: Focused on providing relief from symptoms and stress, palliative care is essential for patients with advanced cancer, addressing their physical, emotional, and spiritual needs.

The Evolving Landscape of Cancer Treatment

The field of oncology is rapidly evolving, driven by advances in research and technology. Genomic profiling and personalized medicine are transforming the way cancer is treated, allowing for tailored therapies that cater to the individual characteristics of a patient's tumor. Ongoing clinical trials continue to investigate new agents, combination therapies, and novel treatment approaches, expanding the arsenal available to oncologists.

Understanding the fundamentals of cancer biology and the various treatment modalities is essential for mastering radiotherapy and chemotherapy. As we delve deeper into the specifics of these treatments in the following chapters, it is crucial to recognize the interconnectedness of these approaches and the significance of a comprehensive, patient-centered strategy in oncology. This knowledge lays the groundwork for navigating the complexities of cancer treatment and optimizing patient outcomes.

With this foundation, we now turn our attention to radiotherapy, exploring its principles, techniques, and applications in the fight against cancer.

Chapter 2: Understanding Radiotherapy

Basics of Radiotherapy

Radiotherapy, also known as radiation therapy, is a cornerstone treatment modality in oncology, utilizing high-energy radiation to kill cancer cells or inhibit their growth. The principle behind radiotherapy is based on the ability of ionizing radiation to damage the DNA of cells, thereby preventing them from replicating and leading to cell death. This chapter delves into the fundamentals of radiotherapy, exploring its types, mechanisms, delivery methods, and clinical applications.

Types of Radiation

Radiotherapy can be broadly categorized into two primary types: **external beam radiotherapy (EBRT)** and **internal radiotherapy (brachytherapy)**. Each type has unique applications and is chosen based on the specific needs of the patient and the characteristics of the cancer being treated.

External Beam Radiotherapy (EBRT)

- **Definition**: EBRT is the most common form of radiotherapy, where high-energy beams (such as X-rays or electrons) are directed at the tumor from outside the body.
- **Mechanism**: The radiation penetrates the body and delivers targeted doses to the tumor while minimizing exposure to surrounding healthy tissues. Modern techniques, such as intensity-modulated radiation therapy (IMRT) and stereotactic radiosurgery (SRS), enhance the precision of radiation delivery, allowing for higher doses to be administered safely.
- **Applications**: EBRT is used in various cancers, including breast, prostate, lung, and brain tumors, often as a curative treatment or as palliative care to relieve symptoms.

Internal Radiotherapy (Brachytherapy)

- **Definition**: Brachytherapy involves placing radioactive sources directly inside or very close to the tumor.
- **Mechanism**: This method allows for a higher dose of radiation to be delivered directly to the tumor with reduced exposure to surrounding healthy tissues. The radiation sources can be permanent (seed implants) or temporary (applicators).
- **Applications**: Brachytherapy is commonly used in cancers of the prostate, cervical, and breast, among others, often as part of a combination treatment strategy.

Mechanisms of Action

The efficacy of radiotherapy lies in its ability to induce DNA damage in cancer cells. This damage can occur through various mechanisms:

- **Direct Ionization**: High-energy radiation can directly ionize the DNA molecules, leading to strand breaks and altering the cellular structure.
- **Indirect Ionization**: Radiation can also ionize water molecules in the body, creating free radicals. These free radicals can then damage DNA, proteins, and cell membranes, contributing to cellular dysfunction and death.

The ability of cancer cells to repair DNA damage varies. Tumors with defective DNA repair mechanisms may be more sensitive to radiation, while those with proficient repair pathways may develop resistance. Understanding these mechanisms informs treatment planning and the potential need for adjunct therapies to enhance radiotherapy's effectiveness.

Application in Cancer Treatment

Radiotherapy is integral to cancer treatment, serving various roles throughout the disease continuum:

1. **Curative Treatment**: In early-stage cancers, radiotherapy may be used as a definitive treatment aimed at eradicating the tumor.
2. **Adjuvant Therapy**: Following surgery, radiotherapy can be employed to eliminate residual cancer cells, reducing the risk of recurrence.
3. **Neoadjuvant Therapy**: Administered before surgery, neoadjuvant radiotherapy can shrink tumors, making them easier to remove surgically.
4. **Palliative Care**: In advanced cancer cases, radiotherapy can alleviate symptoms such as pain, bleeding, or obstruction, improving the quality of life for patients.
5. **Combination with Other Modalities**: Radiotherapy is often used in conjunction with chemotherapy and targeted therapies to enhance treatment outcomes, a strategy known as multimodal therapy.

Treatment Planning in Radiotherapy

Effective radiotherapy relies on meticulous treatment planning. This involves a comprehensive assessment of the patient's cancer type, stage, and overall health, along with precise imaging techniques to define the tumor's size and location. Key components of treatment planning include:

- **Simulation**: Patients undergo imaging (such as CT or MRI) to create a detailed map of the tumor and surrounding tissues, allowing for accurate radiation targeting.
- **Dosimetry**: Calculation of the optimal radiation dose to maximize tumor control while minimizing exposure to healthy tissues. This process involves sophisticated computer algorithms and planning systems.
- **Patient Positioning**: Ensuring the patient is positioned consistently throughout treatment to maintain accuracy in radiation delivery.

Conclusion

Understanding the principles of radiotherapy is essential for mastering its application in cancer treatment. As a powerful tool in the oncologist's arsenal, radiotherapy can significantly impact treatment outcomes, offering curative and palliative options tailored to individual patient needs. In the following chapters, we will explore the intricacies of chemotherapy, its mechanisms, and its integration with radiotherapy to form a comprehensive approach to cancer management.

Chapter 3: Principles of Chemotherapy

Mechanisms of Action

Chemotherapy is a fundamental component of cancer treatment that employs cytotoxic drugs to target and eliminate rapidly dividing cancer cells. The mechanisms by which chemotherapy acts are diverse, reflecting the complexity of cancer biology and the variety of agents available. Understanding these mechanisms is crucial for optimizing treatment regimens and minimizing adverse effects.

Types of Chemotherapy Agents

1. **Alkylating Agents**: These agents work by adding alkyl groups to DNA, leading to cross-linking of DNA strands. This prevents the strands from separating, which is necessary for DNA replication and transcription. Alkylating agents are effective against various cancers, including lymphoma and leukemia.

2. **Antimetabolites**: These drugs mimic the building blocks of DNA and RNA, interfering with the synthesis of nucleic acids. By incorporating into the DNA or RNA, they disrupt the normal cellular processes of replication and repair. Common examples include methotrexate and 5-fluorouracil, often used in cancers such as breast and colon cancer.

3. **Antitumor Antibiotics**: These are not like traditional antibiotics; they specifically target cancer cells. They bind to DNA, preventing the synthesis of nucleic acids. Doxorubicin and bleomycin are notable examples, used in various cancers, including breast cancer and Hodgkin lymphoma.

4. **Topoisomerase Inhibitors**: These agents interfere with the enzymes that help unwind DNA for replication. By blocking these enzymes, they induce DNA breaks, ultimately leading to cell death. Examples include etoposide and irinotecan, used in lung cancer and colorectal cancer.

5. **Mitotic Inhibitors**: Derived from natural sources like the periwinkle plant, these drugs disrupt the microtubule structures necessary for cell division. Paclitaxel and vincristine are common examples, often used in breast cancer and leukemia.

Chemotherapy agents can be categorized based on their chemical structure, mechanism of action, and the cancer types they target. This categorization is essential for tailoring treatment regimens:

1. **Cytotoxic Chemotherapy**: This includes the majority of traditional chemotherapy drugs that kill or inhibit the growth of cancer cells. These agents are typically non-specific, affecting both cancerous and normal cells.
2. **Targeted Therapy**: Unlike cytotoxic chemotherapy, targeted therapies focus on specific molecular targets associated with cancer. These drugs are designed to interfere with specific pathways crucial for tumor growth and survival. Examples include trastuzumab (Herceptin) for HER2-positive breast cancer and imatinib (Gleevec) for chronic myeloid leukemia.
3. **Hormonal Therapy**: Hormonal therapies block the body's natural hormones from supporting the growth of cancer. This approach is particularly effective in cancers like breast and prostate cancer, where hormone receptors play a significant role. Tamoxifen and aromatase inhibitors are commonly used in breast cancer management.
4. **Immunotherapy**: This innovative approach harnesses the body's immune system to fight cancer. Immune checkpoint inhibitors (e.g., pembrolizumab and nivolumab) enhance the immune response against cancer cells and are increasingly used across various malignancies.

Roles in Cancer Management

Chemotherapy plays several critical roles in cancer management, which can vary depending on the cancer type, stage, and patient factors. Understanding these roles is vital for effective treatment planning:

1. **Curative Intent**: In some cases, chemotherapy can eliminate cancer entirely, especially when used in combination with other modalities such as surgery or radiotherapy.
2. **Adjuvant Therapy**: Chemotherapy is often administered post-surgery to eliminate residual disease and reduce the risk of recurrence. This is particularly common in breast, colon, and ovarian cancers.
3. **Neoadjuvant Therapy**: When chemotherapy is given before surgery, it can shrink tumors, making them more operable. This approach is frequently used in locally advanced breast and bladder cancers.
4. **Palliative Care**: In advanced cancer cases, chemotherapy may be used to relieve symptoms and improve quality of life, even if curative treatment is not possible. This palliative approach is vital for enhancing patient comfort.
5. **Maintenance Therapy**: For some cancers, ongoing chemotherapy may be used to keep the disease in remission after an initial response, aiming to prolong survival and manage symptoms.

Administration of Chemotherapy

Chemotherapy can be administered through various routes, including intravenous (IV), oral, intramuscular, subcutaneous, and even intrathecal (directly into the spinal fluid). The route of administration often depends on the specific drug, the treatment goals, and the patient's overall health.

1. **Intravenous Administration**: The most common method, allowing for immediate systemic distribution of the drug. IV chemotherapy can be delivered in outpatient settings or hospital environments, depending on the regimen.
2. **Oral Chemotherapy**: Some chemotherapy agents are available in pill form, offering convenience and the ability for patients to take their medication at home. However, careful monitoring is required to ensure adherence and manage side effects.
3. **Combination Therapy**: Often, multiple agents are used together to maximize efficacy and minimize resistance. The selection of drugs is based on the cancer type, genetic factors, and previous treatment history.

Conclusion

Understanding the principles of chemotherapy, including its mechanisms of action and various types of agents, is essential for mastering its application in cancer management. As we continue this journey through the intricacies of cancer treatment, the next chapter will focus on treatment planning in radiotherapy, outlining the key components involved in creating effective and personalized treatment strategies for patients. This foundation will further enhance our ability to integrate chemotherapy with radiotherapy and other modalities for optimal cancer care.

Chapter 4: Treatment Planning in Radiotherapy
Key Components of Treatment Planning

Effective treatment planning in radiotherapy is crucial for maximizing the therapeutic benefits of radiation while minimizing damage to surrounding healthy tissues. A comprehensive treatment plan involves several key components, including patient simulation, dosimetry, and precise patient positioning. Each element plays a vital role in ensuring that radiation is delivered accurately and safely.

1. Patient Simulation

Patient simulation is the first step in the treatment planning process. This phase involves creating a detailed representation of the patient's anatomy, which will guide the radiation delivery system.

- **Imaging Techniques**: Advanced imaging modalities such as computed tomography (CT), magnetic resonance imaging (MRI), and positron emission tomography (PET) are used to visualize the tumor and surrounding structures. These images provide critical information about the tumor's size, shape, and location, which is essential for accurate treatment planning.
- **Immobilization**: During simulation, patients may be placed in custom-made devices to ensure they remain in the same position for each treatment session. This immobilization is critical for achieving consistent and precise radiation delivery.
- **Simulation Process**: The simulation typically involves positioning the patient on a treatment couch and obtaining images in the planned treatment position. Markers or tattoos may be used on the patient's skin to identify the treatment area consistently.

2. Dosimetry

Dosimetry refers to the calculation and measurement of the radiation dose that will be delivered to the tumor and surrounding tissues.

- **Treatment Planning Systems (TPS)**: Modern TPS use sophisticated algorithms to determine the optimal radiation dose distribution. These systems analyze the imaging data from the simulation phase to calculate the appropriate doses needed to effectively target the tumor while sparing healthy tissue.
- **Dose Prescription**: The oncologist specifies the total dose and fractionation schedule (the number of treatment sessions and the dose delivered each session) based on the type of cancer, its stage, and the patient's overall health. This prescription is crucial for ensuring that the radiation is delivered effectively over time.
- **Verification**: Prior to the initiation of treatment, dosimetric calculations are verified through various quality assurance processes. These may include comparing planned doses against delivered doses using phantom studies or advanced dosimeters.

3. Patient Positioning

Precise patient positioning is fundamental to successful radiotherapy.

- **Consistency**: Maintaining the same patient position for each treatment session is crucial. Variations in position can lead to suboptimal radiation delivery, potentially reducing treatment effectiveness and increasing the risk of side effects.
- **Positioning Devices**: Various devices, such as cushions, molds, and boards, are employed to keep patients in the correct position. These aids help stabilize the patient and prevent movement during treatment.
- **Verification Imaging**: Before each treatment session, imaging techniques such as cone-beam CT (CBCT) may be used to confirm that the patient is correctly positioned. If discrepancies are detected, adjustments can be made to ensure accurate delivery of the radiation dose.

4. Treatment Delivery

Once the treatment plan is finalized, the next step is the delivery of radiation to the patient.

- **Linear Accelerators (Linacs)**: Most radiotherapy treatments are delivered using linear accelerators, which generate high-energy X-rays or electrons. These machines are equipped with advanced imaging systems that assist in verifying patient positioning before treatment.
- **Treatment Techniques**: Several techniques may be utilized, including conventional radiation therapy, intensity-modulated radiation therapy (IMRT), volumetric modulated arc therapy (VMAT), and stereotactic body radiation therapy (SBRT). The choice of technique depends on the tumor type, location, and specific treatment goals.

5. Quality Assurance and Safety

Ensuring the safety and accuracy of the treatment delivery process is paramount.

- **Quality Assurance Programs**: Comprehensive quality assurance (QA) programs are implemented to regularly check the calibration of radiation delivery systems, verify treatment plans, and monitor patient safety. These QA measures help prevent errors and enhance treatment outcomes.
- **Patient Monitoring**: During treatment, patients are monitored for any immediate side effects or complications. Effective communication between patients and healthcare providers is crucial to address any concerns promptly.

Conclusion

Treatment planning in radiotherapy is a multifaceted process that requires careful consideration of patient-specific factors, advanced imaging techniques, and precise dosimetry. Each component, from simulation to patient positioning and treatment delivery, is integral to achieving optimal treatment outcomes while minimizing harm to healthy tissues. As we continue our exploration of cancer treatment, the next chapter will focus on chemotherapy protocols, examining common regimens used for various cancer types and their administration guidelines. This knowledge will further enhance our understanding of how radiotherapy and chemotherapy can be effectively integrated for comprehensive cancer care.

Chapter 5: Chemotherapy Protocols

Common Chemotherapy Regimens for Various Cancer Types and Their Administration Guidelines

Chemotherapy is a critical component of cancer treatment, often utilized in various settings—curative, adjuvant, neoadjuvant, and palliative. Understanding common chemotherapy regimens, their administration protocols, and the specific cancer types they target is essential for effectively managing patient care. This chapter outlines several key regimens used for various cancers, along with guidelines for their administration.

1. Breast Cancer

Common Regimens:

- **AC (Adriamycin and Cyclophosphamide)**: Administered every three weeks for four cycles. Doxorubicin (Adriamycin) and cyclophosphamide are given intravenously. This regimen is often followed by taxane-based therapy (e.g., paclitaxel).
- **TC (Docetaxel and Cyclophosphamide)**: Administered every three weeks for four cycles. This combination is used for patients with node-positive breast cancer.

Administration Guidelines:

- Monitor cardiac function before and during treatment due to the cardiotoxicity associated with doxorubicin.
- Supportive medications, including antiemetics, should be administered to manage side effects such as nausea.

2. Lung Cancer

Common Regimens:

- **Cisplatin-based Regimens**: A common choice for non-small cell lung cancer (NSCLC). Typical combinations include cisplatin with pemetrexed (Alimta) or docetaxel, administered every three weeks.
- **Carboplatin with Paclitaxel**: Often used in patients with advanced NSCLC. The carboplatin dose is calculated based on the patient's renal function, using the Calvert formula.

Administration Guidelines:

- Pre-medication with antiemetics is critical due to the high incidence of nausea and vomiting.
- Regular monitoring of renal function is important due to the nephrotoxicity of cisplatin and carboplatin.

3. Colorectal Cancer

Common Regimens:

- **FOLFOX (Fluorouracil, Leucovorin, and Oxaliplatin)**: Administered every two weeks. Leucovorin enhances the efficacy of fluorouracil, while oxaliplatin adds additional anti-cancer activity.
- **FOLFIRI (Fluorouracil, Leucovorin, and Irinotecan)**: Also administered every two weeks. This regimen is commonly used for patients with metastatic disease.

Administration Guidelines:

- Monitor for neuropathy due to oxaliplatin and adjust doses accordingly.
- Manage diarrhea, especially with irinotecan, by providing loperamide as needed.

4. Ovarian Cancer

Common Regimens:

- **Carboplatin and Paclitaxel**: This combination is typically administered every three weeks for six cycles. This regimen is standard for newly diagnosed ovarian cancer.
- **Dose-Dense Paclitaxel**: Paclitaxel is given weekly for the first 18 weeks in combination with carboplatin.

Administration Guidelines:

- Pre-medication with corticosteroids and antihistamines is necessary to reduce allergic reactions associated with paclitaxel.
- Regular blood counts should be monitored to manage myelosuppression risks.

5. Lymphoma

Common Regimens:

- **CHOP (Cyclophosphamide, Doxorubicin, Vincristine, and Prednisone)**: Administered every three weeks for six to eight cycles. CHOP is commonly used for non-Hodgkin lymphoma.
- **R-CHOP**: Incorporates rituximab with the CHOP regimen for CD20-positive lymphomas.

Administration Guidelines:

- Monitor for cardiac and liver function due to the potential toxicities of doxorubicin and cyclophosphamide.
- Provide prophylaxis for tumor lysis syndrome in high-risk patients.

6. Bladder Cancer

Common Regimens:

- **Gemcitabine and Cisplatin**: Administered every three weeks for muscle-invasive bladder cancer.
- **MVAC (Methotrexate, Vinblastine, Doxorubicin, and Cisplatin)**: An alternative regimen, administered every three weeks.

Administration Guidelines:

- Hydration and diuresis are essential to reduce the risk of cisplatin nephrotoxicity.
- Monitor electrolyte levels and renal function during treatment.

7. Administration Guidelines for Chemotherapy

- **Patient Education**: It is vital to educate patients about the treatment regimen, potential side effects, and the importance of adherence to appointments.
- **Supportive Care**: Integrate supportive measures, including antiemetics, growth factors, and nutritional support, to enhance patient comfort and treatment efficacy.
- **Monitoring**: Regular follow-up visits are essential for assessing treatment response, managing side effects, and adjusting doses as needed.

Conclusion

Chemotherapy protocols are integral to cancer management, offering various options tailored to the specific needs of patients based on their cancer type and overall health. Understanding these regimens, their administration guidelines, and the accompanying supportive care strategies is crucial for optimizing treatment outcomes. In the following chapter, we will discuss the side effects of radiotherapy, including acute and chronic effects, and explore strategies for their management to enhance patient care throughout the treatment journey.

Chapter 6: Side Effects of Radiotherapy
Discussing Acute and Chronic Side Effects and Their Management Strategies

Radiotherapy is a powerful tool in the fight against cancer, but like any medical intervention, it comes with potential side effects. Understanding these effects—both acute and chronic—is crucial for patients and healthcare providers alike. This chapter explores the nature of these side effects, their underlying mechanisms, and effective management strategies to improve patient outcomes and quality of life.

1. Acute Side Effects

Acute side effects are those that occur during or shortly after treatment, typically within days to weeks. These effects are often temporary but can significantly impact a patient's well-being during the treatment course.

Common Acute Side Effects:

Skin Reactions

Management

- Patients should be advised to keep the skin clean and moisturized, using mild soaps and emollients.
- Avoidance of tight clothing, heat, and direct sun exposure to the treated area is recommended.

Fatigue

Management

- Encourage patients to engage in light physical activity, such as walking, to help combat fatigue.
- Adequate rest and a balanced diet can also support energy levels.

Nausea and Vomiting

Management

- Prophylactic antiemetics should be administered prior to treatment to reduce nausea.
- Dietary modifications, such as small, frequent meals, can help alleviate symptoms.

Mucositis

Management

- Use of saline rinses, topical anesthetics, and oral care products can provide relief.
- A diet of soft foods and increased hydration may also be beneficial.

2. Chronic Side Effects

Chronic side effects can emerge months or even years after treatment. These may result from cumulative damage to healthy tissues during radiation exposure and can significantly impact a patient's long-term quality of life.

Common Chronic Side Effects:

Fibrosis

Management

- Physical therapy and rehabilitation exercises can help maintain flexibility and strength.
- In some cases, surgical interventions may be necessary.

Lymphedema

Management

- Early referral to a lymphedema specialist for compression therapy, manual lymphatic drainage, and exercise.
- Patient education on self-care techniques is vital.

Secondary Cancers

Management

- Long-term follow-up and surveillance are essential to detect any new cancers early.
- Encourage lifestyle modifications, such as smoking cessation and healthy diet, to reduce cancer risk.

Cognitive Changes

Management

- Neuropsychological evaluations and cognitive rehabilitation programs can assist affected patients.
- Support groups and educational resources can help patients and families navigate these changes.

3. Psychological Impact

In addition to physical side effects, the psychological impact of radiotherapy should not be overlooked. Patients may experience anxiety, depression, or changes in body image.

Management Strategies:

- **Psychological Support**: Referral to mental health professionals for counseling or support groups can provide patients with coping strategies and emotional support.
- **Patient Education**: Providing clear information about what to expect during treatment can reduce anxiety and help patients feel more in control.

Conclusion

The side effects of radiotherapy can vary widely among patients, and effective management is essential for maintaining quality of life during and after treatment. Understanding both acute and chronic side effects allows healthcare providers to implement proactive strategies that enhance patient comfort and treatment adherence.

In the next chapter, we will explore how to manage chemotherapy side effects, building upon the knowledge gained in this chapter to provide a comprehensive overview of supportive care in cancer treatment. By addressing the side effects associated with both radiotherapy and chemotherapy, we can improve overall treatment experiences and outcomes for patients facing cancer.

Chapter 7: Managing Chemotherapy Side Effects

Overview of Common Side Effects of Chemotherapy and Supportive Care Options

Chemotherapy, while an effective treatment modality for many cancers, often comes with a range of side effects that can significantly impact a patient's quality of life. Understanding these side effects and implementing effective management strategies is critical for enhancing patient comfort and compliance with treatment regimens. This chapter outlines common chemotherapy side effects and offers supportive care options to alleviate these challenges.

1. Common Side Effects of Chemotherapy

Chemotherapy can cause both acute and chronic side effects. The nature and severity of these effects vary based on the specific drugs used, the patient's individual characteristics, and the cancer being treated.

Common Acute Side Effects:

- **Nausea and Vomiting**: One of the most distressing side effects of chemotherapy, nausea and vomiting can occur shortly after treatment and may persist for several days. The severity can vary depending on the specific drugs used.
- **Fatigue**: Many patients experience fatigue, which can be exacerbated by the physical and emotional stress of a cancer diagnosis and treatment. This fatigue may not be relieved by rest and can impact daily activities.
- **Myelosuppression**: This refers to the decreased production of blood cells in the bone marrow, leading to anemia, increased risk of infections (due to low white blood cell counts), and a tendency to bleed or bruise easily (due to low platelet counts).
- **Mucositis**: Inflammation and ulceration of the mucous membranes, particularly in the mouth and gastrointestinal tract, can result in painful sores and difficulty swallowing or eating.
- **Alopecia**: Hair loss is a common side effect of many chemotherapeutic agents, which can have a significant psychological impact on patients.

Common Chronic Side Effects:

- **Peripheral Neuropathy**: Some chemotherapy agents, particularly platinum-based drugs and taxanes, can cause nerve damage, leading to tingling, numbness, or pain in the hands and feet.
- **Cognitive Changes**: Patients may experience cognitive difficulties, often referred to as "chemo brain," characterized by problems with memory, attention, and processing speed.
- **Long-term Fatigue**: For some patients, fatigue can persist long after treatment has ended, affecting their overall quality of life.
- **Secondary Malignancies**: There is a risk of developing secondary cancers, particularly after certain chemotherapeutic regimens, which may necessitate ongoing monitoring.

2. Supportive Care Options

Managing the side effects of chemotherapy requires a proactive and multifaceted approach. Here are key strategies to mitigate common side effects:

Nausea and Vomiting:

- **Antiemetic Medications**: Prophylactic use of antiemetics, such as ondansetron or granisetron, can significantly reduce the incidence of nausea and vomiting. Regimens may be tailored based on the emetogenic potential of the chemotherapy agent.
- **Dietary Modifications**: Encourage patients to consume small, frequent meals that are bland and easy to digest. Ginger and peppermint may also provide relief.

Fatigue:

- **Exercise**: Encouraging light to moderate exercise, such as walking, can help alleviate fatigue and improve overall well-being.
- **Rest and Sleep Hygiene**: Establishing a routine for rest and practicing good sleep hygiene can enhance energy levels.

Myelosuppression:

- **Regular Blood Counts**: Monitoring blood counts helps to identify and address myelosuppression early.
- **Growth Factors**: Agents such as filgrastim (G-CSF) can stimulate white blood cell production and reduce the risk of infection.
- **Transfusions**: In cases of severe anemia or thrombocytopenia, blood transfusions may be necessary.

Mucositis:

- **Oral Care Protocols**: Encourage frequent oral hygiene practices, including using gentle mouth rinses (e.g., saline or baking soda solutions) and avoiding irritants such as alcohol and tobacco.
- **Topical Agents**: The use of topical anesthetics or protective oral coatings can alleviate pain associated with mucositis.

Alopecia:

- **Wigs and Head Coverings**: Providing resources and support for patients considering wigs or head coverings can help address the psychosocial impact of hair loss.
- **Scalp Cooling**: Some patients may benefit from scalp cooling systems during chemotherapy to reduce the risk of hair loss.

Peripheral Neuropathy:

- **Early Intervention**: Patients should be educated to report symptoms early, allowing for timely interventions or dose adjustments.
- **Medications**: Medications such as gabapentin or duloxetine may be prescribed to manage neuropathic pain.

Cognitive Changes:

- **Cognitive Rehabilitation**: Referral to cognitive rehabilitation programs can help patients develop strategies to cope with cognitive challenges.
- **Education and Support**: Providing information about the potential for cognitive changes can help patients manage their expectations and seek appropriate support.

Conclusion

Effectively managing the side effects of chemotherapy is essential for enhancing patient comfort and adherence to treatment protocols. By understanding the common side effects and implementing supportive care strategies, healthcare providers can significantly improve the quality of life for patients undergoing chemotherapy.

In the next chapter, we will explore the rationale and strategies for combining therapies, specifically focusing on how radiotherapy and chemotherapy can be integrated to optimize cancer treatment outcomes. This integrated approach can provide a comprehensive framework for addressing the complexities of cancer management and improving patient care.

Chapter 8: Combining Therapies: Radiotherapy and Chemotherapy

Rationale and Strategies for Combining Treatments

The integration of radiotherapy and chemotherapy represents a pivotal advancement in cancer treatment, leveraging the strengths of both modalities to enhance therapeutic effectiveness and improve patient outcomes. This chapter explores the rationale behind combining these therapies, the various strategies employed, and the clinical implications of such approaches.

1. Rationale for Combination Therapy

Combining radiotherapy and chemotherapy is based on several principles that capitalize on the complementary effects of each treatment modality:

- **Enhanced Tumor Control**: Radiotherapy primarily targets localized tumors, while chemotherapy acts systemically. By combining the two, clinicians aim to eradicate cancer cells in both the primary tumor and any potential metastatic sites.
- **Improved Response Rates**: Studies have shown that the concurrent administration of chemotherapy can sensitize cancer cells to radiation, making them more susceptible to damage. This is particularly effective in rapidly dividing cells, which are characteristic of many cancers.
- **Decreased Risk of Recurrence**: By using both treatments, the likelihood of residual cancer cells surviving post-treatment is reduced, potentially lowering the risk of local and distant recurrences.
- **Synergistic Effects**: Certain chemotherapeutic agents can enhance the effects of radiation therapy. For example, agents that cause DNA damage or inhibit DNA repair can amplify the cytotoxic effects of radiotherapy.

2. Strategies for Combining Treatments

Combining radiotherapy and chemotherapy can be approached in several ways, depending on the specific cancer type, treatment goals, and patient characteristics.

Concurrent Therapy:

- In concurrent therapy, chemotherapy and radiotherapy are administered simultaneously, either during the same treatment cycle or on alternating days.
- **Indications**: This approach is commonly used in locally advanced cancers such as head and neck, cervical, and lung cancers.
- **Benefits**: Concurrent therapy can enhance local control and improve overall survival rates compared to sequential therapies.
- **Challenges**: Increased toxicity is a concern, as patients may experience exacerbated side effects from both treatments, requiring careful management and supportive care.

Sequential Therapy:

- Sequential therapy involves administering chemotherapy and radiotherapy in a staged manner, where one modality follows the other.
- **Indications**: This approach may be employed in situations where the tumor burden is initially reduced with chemotherapy before radiotherapy is applied.
- **Example**: Neoadjuvant chemotherapy may be given before surgery and followed by adjuvant radiotherapy to eliminate residual disease.
- **Benefits**: Sequential therapy can allow for better tolerance of each treatment, as patients may recover from one before starting the next.

Combination in Palliative Care:

- In patients with advanced cancer, combining radiotherapy and chemotherapy may be aimed at palliative care to alleviate symptoms.
- **Example**: Palliative radiotherapy can be combined with systemic chemotherapy to relieve pain from metastatic lesions while also targeting cancer control.

3. Clinical Considerations

While combining radiotherapy and chemotherapy can be highly effective, several clinical considerations must be addressed:

- **Patient Selection**: Not all patients are suitable candidates for combined therapy. Factors such as tumor type, stage, patient comorbidities, and overall performance status must be evaluated.
- **Timing and Scheduling**: The timing of administering chemotherapy in relation to radiotherapy is crucial. Optimizing the schedule to maximize synergistic effects while minimizing toxicity requires careful planning and coordination among the oncology team.
- **Monitoring and Management of Side Effects**: The combination of therapies may lead to increased side effects. Ongoing assessment and prompt management of adverse events are essential to maintain quality of life and adherence to treatment.
- **Interdisciplinary Collaboration**: Successful implementation of combined therapy necessitates a multidisciplinary approach, involving oncologists, radiologists, nurses, and supportive care providers to ensure comprehensive patient management.

4. Case Examples of Combined Therapy

- **Head and Neck Cancer**: In locally advanced head and neck squamous cell carcinoma, concurrent chemoradiotherapy with cisplatin has shown improved survival rates compared to radiotherapy alone.
- **Cervical Cancer**: The use of concurrent chemoradiotherapy in locally advanced cervical cancer has become the standard of care, resulting in enhanced local control and improved overall survival.
- **Lung Cancer**: For stage III non-small cell lung cancer, combining chemotherapy with concurrent radiation has significantly improved outcomes, although it comes with increased toxicity.

Conclusion

Combining radiotherapy and chemotherapy presents a powerful strategy in the fight against cancer, allowing for enhanced tumor control and improved patient outcomes. Understanding the rationale for such combinations, the various strategies employed, and the clinical considerations involved is essential for optimizing cancer treatment.

In the next chapter, we will explore the advances in radiotherapy techniques, including emerging technologies such as IMRT, SRS, and SBRT, and their impact on treatment outcomes. By understanding these advancements, healthcare providers can continue to improve the precision and effectiveness of cancer therapies.

Chapter 9: Advances in Radiotherapy Techniques

Emerging Technologies: IMRT, SRS, and SBRT, and Their Impact on Treatment Outcomes

Radiotherapy has undergone significant advancements over the past few decades, transforming how cancer is treated. Innovations in technology have led to more precise delivery of radiation, allowing for higher doses to be administered safely while minimizing damage to surrounding healthy tissues. This chapter explores three key advances in radiotherapy techniques—Intensity-Modulated Radiation Therapy (IMRT), Stereotactic Radiosurgery (SRS), and Stereotactic Body Radiation Therapy (SBRT)—and their impact on treatment outcomes.

1. Intensity-Modulated Radiation Therapy (IMRT)

Overview:

IMRT is a sophisticated form of radiotherapy that allows for the modulation of radiation intensity across different parts of the treatment field. By using advanced computer algorithms and imaging techniques, IMRT can deliver varying doses of radiation to different areas within the tumor, sparing healthy tissues and organs at risk.

Technical Aspects:

- **Multileaf Collimator (MLC)**: IMRT employs a multileaf collimator to shape the radiation beam precisely, enabling it to conform to the tumor's three-dimensional shape.
- **Dose Optimization**: Treatment planning systems (TPS) calculate the optimal radiation distribution, taking into account the tumor's location, size, and proximity to critical structures.

Clinical Applications:

IMRT is particularly beneficial for cancers located near critical organs, such as head and neck cancers, prostate cancer, and breast cancer. It reduces the risk of radiation-related complications, such as xerostomia (dry mouth) in head and neck cancer patients and rectal toxicity in prostate cancer patients.

Impact on Treatment Outcomes:

Clinical studies have demonstrated that IMRT can improve local control rates, reduce treatment-related side effects, and enhance overall quality of life for patients. Patients often report better functional outcomes and reduced incidence of complications compared to conventional radiotherapy.

2. Stereotactic Radiosurgery (SRS)

Overview:

Stereotactic radiosurgery is a non-invasive procedure that delivers high doses of radiation precisely to targeted tumors, often in a single session. SRS is commonly used for treating brain tumors, arteriovenous malformations (AVMs), and metastatic lesions in the brain.

Technical Aspects:

- **Frame-Based or Frameless Systems**: SRS can be performed using a rigid frame to stabilize the patient's head or frameless systems that utilize advanced imaging techniques for precise localization.
- **High-Precision Targeting**: Utilizing multiple beams converging on the tumor, SRS minimizes exposure to surrounding healthy tissues while delivering a potent dose to the tumor.

Clinical Applications:

SRS is particularly effective for small to medium-sized brain tumors and is often preferred for patients who are not surgical candidates due to health concerns.

Impact on Treatment Outcomes:

Studies indicate that SRS can achieve high rates of tumor control with minimal side effects. For many patients, SRS can effectively halt tumor growth, improve survival rates, and enhance quality of life compared to traditional surgery.

3. Stereotactic Body Radiation Therapy (SBRT)

Overview:

SBRT is a technique similar to SRS but applied to tumors located outside the brain, such as those in the lung, liver, pancreas, and spine. It involves delivering very high doses of radiation in a few treatment sessions, typically ranging from one to five.

Technical Aspects:

- **Advanced Imaging**: SBRT relies on precise imaging techniques such as CT and MRI to accurately locate tumors and track patient movement during treatment.
- **Real-Time Tracking**: Techniques like respiratory gating help account for tumor movement during breathing, ensuring accurate radiation delivery.

Clinical Applications:

SBRT is effective for early-stage lung cancer, oligometastatic disease, and certain primary tumors. Its ability to deliver high doses over fewer sessions is particularly advantageous for patients who may struggle with prolonged treatment courses.

Impact on Treatment Outcomes:

Research shows that SBRT can achieve excellent local control rates with a favorable safety profile. It allows for aggressive treatment of tumors while minimizing damage to adjacent healthy tissues, resulting in improved patient outcomes and quality of life.

4. Conclusion

Advances in radiotherapy techniques, including IMRT, SRS, and SBRT, represent significant milestones in cancer treatment. These technologies enhance the precision of radiation delivery, improve treatment outcomes, and reduce side effects. As these techniques continue to evolve, they hold the potential to further refine cancer treatment and improve patient experiences.

In the next chapter, we will explore novel chemotherapy agents and targeted therapies, examining how these developments complement advances in radiotherapy. By understanding the interplay between these treatment modalities, healthcare providers can enhance their approach to comprehensive cancer care.

Chapter 10: Novel Chemotherapy Agents and Targeted Therapy

Exploration of New Drug Classes, Targeted Therapies, and Immunotherapy in Cancer Treatment

The landscape of chemotherapy is continually evolving, driven by advancements in research and technology. Novel chemotherapy agents and targeted therapies have emerged as vital components of cancer treatment, offering new hope for patients and expanding the therapeutic arsenal available to oncologists. This chapter delves into the various classes of novel agents, the principles of targeted therapy, and the exciting developments in immunotherapy.

1. Novel Chemotherapy Agents

Recent years have seen the introduction of several new chemotherapy agents that demonstrate improved efficacy and reduced toxicity compared to traditional cytotoxic drugs. These agents can be classified into several categories based on their mechanisms of action.

a. Antibody-Drug Conjugates (ADCs):

- ADCs combine the specificity of monoclonal antibodies with the potent cytotoxicity of chemotherapy agents. By linking a cytotoxic drug to an antibody that targets a specific tumor antigen, ADCs can deliver treatment directly to cancer cells while minimizing damage to healthy tissues.
- **Example**: Trastuzumab emtansine (Kadcyla) is an ADC used in HER2-positive breast cancer, delivering a potent chemotherapy agent directly to cells expressing HER2.

b. Poly(ADP-ribose) Polymerase (PARP) Inhibitors:

- PARP inhibitors target cancer cells with defective DNA repair mechanisms, particularly those with BRCA1 or BRCA2 mutations. By inhibiting the PARP enzyme, these drugs prevent cancer cells from repairing DNA damage, leading to cell death.
- **Example**: Olaparib (Lynparza) is a PARP inhibitor approved for use in ovarian and breast cancers associated with BRCA mutations.

c. Immune Checkpoint Inhibitors (though primarily immunotherapy, some act as chemotherapy):

- While not traditional chemotherapy, immune checkpoint inhibitors are revolutionizing cancer treatment by enhancing the immune response against tumors. These agents target proteins that inhibit immune activation, effectively unleashing the body's immune system to attack cancer cells.
- **Example**: Pembrolizumab (Keytruda) and nivolumab (Opdivo) target PD-1 and have shown effectiveness in various cancers, including melanoma, lung cancer, and bladder cancer.

2. Targeted Therapy

Targeted therapies are designed to specifically attack cancer cells based on their molecular characteristics, allowing for more personalized treatment strategies. These therapies typically focus on specific genetic mutations, proteins, or pathways involved in cancer progression.

a. Tyrosine Kinase Inhibitors (TKIs):

- TKIs block specific enzymes (tyrosine kinases) involved in signaling pathways that promote cancer cell growth and proliferation. By inhibiting these pathways, TKIs can effectively reduce tumor growth.
- **Example**: Imatinib (Gleevec) is a TKI used to treat chronic myeloid leukemia (CML) and gastrointestinal stromal tumors (GISTs) by targeting the BCR-ABL fusion protein.

b. Monoclonal Antibodies:

- These lab-engineered antibodies can specifically target cancer cells or proteins in the tumor microenvironment. Monoclonal antibodies can either directly kill cancer cells, mark them for destruction by the immune system, or inhibit their growth by blocking signaling pathways.
- **Example**: Rituximab (Rituxan) targets CD20 on B-cells and is used in the treatment of non-Hodgkin lymphoma and chronic lymphocytic leukemia.

c. Proteasome Inhibitors:

- Proteasome inhibitors disrupt the protein degradation pathway that is essential for cancer cell survival. By preventing the breakdown of regulatory proteins, these agents can induce apoptosis in malignant cells.
- **Example**: Bortezomib (Velcade) is used in multiple myeloma and certain types of lymphoma, demonstrating significant efficacy in clinical settings.

3. Immunotherapy

Immunotherapy represents a paradigm shift in cancer treatment, leveraging the body's immune system to recognize and destroy cancer cells. This approach can be particularly effective for tumors that are resistant to traditional therapies.

a. Checkpoint Inhibitors:

As mentioned, checkpoint inhibitors like pembrolizumab and nivolumab enhance the immune response by blocking inhibitory signals that prevent T-cells from attacking cancer cells. These agents have transformed the treatment of melanoma, lung cancer, and others.

b. CAR T-Cell Therapy:

- Chimeric antigen receptor (CAR) T-cell therapy involves modifying a patient's T-cells to express a receptor that targets specific cancer antigens. Once reintroduced into the patient, these engineered T-cells can effectively target and kill cancer cells.
- **Example**: CAR T-cell therapies like axicabtagene ciloleucel (Yescarta) have shown remarkable success in treating certain types of B-cell lymphomas.

c. Cancer Vaccines:

- Cancer vaccines aim to stimulate an immune response against specific cancer antigens. While still largely in the investigational stage, several vaccines are being evaluated in clinical trials.
- **Example**: Sipuleucel-T (Provenge) is an approved therapeutic vaccine for prostate cancer that trains the immune system to target prostate cancer cells.

4. Conclusion

The development of novel chemotherapy agents and targeted therapies is transforming the landscape of cancer treatment, providing more effective and less toxic options for patients. Advances in immunotherapy are further enhancing treatment possibilities, allowing for personalized and precision approaches to cancer care.

As we continue to learn more about the molecular underpinnings of cancer, the integration of these novel therapies with traditional treatments like radiotherapy and chemotherapy will play a crucial role in improving patient outcomes. In the next chapter, we will explore the role of genomic profiling in personalizing treatment, highlighting how molecular diagnostics can tailor radiotherapy and chemotherapy to individual patients. This approach will pave the way for more targeted and effective cancer therapies in the future.

Chapter 11: Personalizing Treatment: Genomic Profiling
The Role of Molecular Diagnostics in Tailoring Radiotherapy and Chemotherapy to Individual Patients

As cancer research continues to evolve, the understanding of cancer at the molecular level has led to significant advancements in treatment strategies. Genomic profiling, a crucial component of precision medicine, enables the customization of treatment plans based on the unique genetic makeup of a patient's tumor. This chapter explores the principles of genomic profiling, its applications in personalizing cancer treatment, and its impact on the efficacy of radiotherapy and chemotherapy.

1. Understanding Genomic Profiling

Genomic profiling involves analyzing the genetic alterations within tumor cells to identify mutations, amplifications, deletions, and other genomic changes that drive cancer development and progression. This process typically employs next-generation sequencing (NGS) technologies, which allow for the rapid and comprehensive analysis of multiple genes simultaneously.

Key Components of Genomic Profiling:

- **Targeted Panels**: These panels focus on specific sets of genes known to be involved in particular cancer types. For example, breast cancer panels may target the BRCA1, BRCA2, and HER2 genes.
- **Whole Exome Sequencing (WES)**: This approach sequences all the protein-coding regions of the genome, providing a more extensive overview of potential mutations.
- **Whole Genome Sequencing (WGS)**: While more comprehensive than WES, WGS examines the entire genome, including non-coding regions, offering deeper insights into genomic alterations that may contribute to cancer.

2. Applications of Genomic Profiling in Cancer Treatment

Genomic profiling provides valuable insights that can guide treatment decisions, including:

a. Identification of Targetable Mutations:

Many cancers exhibit specific mutations that can be targeted by available therapies. For instance, patients with non-small cell lung cancer (NSCLC) may benefit from targeted therapies like osimertinib if they possess an EGFR mutation.

b. Predicting Treatment Response:

Genomic alterations can help predict how well a patient will respond to certain treatments. For example, the presence of a specific mutation may indicate a likelihood of benefiting from a particular chemotherapy regimen or targeted therapy.

c. Assessing Prognosis:

Some genomic signatures can provide prognostic information, helping to stratify patients based on their risk of recurrence or progression. This knowledge can inform treatment intensity and monitoring strategies.

d. Tailoring Radiotherapy:

Genomic profiling can influence radiotherapy decisions by identifying tumors with specific characteristics that may be more or less sensitive to radiation. For example, tumors with defects in DNA repair mechanisms may respond better to radiotherapy, allowing for more aggressive treatment approaches.

3. Case Examples of Genomic Profiling in Action

- **Breast Cancer**: Genomic profiling has revolutionized the treatment of breast cancer, particularly through the use of Oncotype DX and MammaPrint tests. These tests assess the expression of specific genes to predict the risk of recurrence and the potential benefit of chemotherapy in early-stage hormone receptor-positive breast cancer. Based on these results, patients may avoid unnecessary chemotherapy.
- **Colorectal Cancer**: The identification of KRAS and NRAS mutations in colorectal cancer has significant implications for treatment. Patients with wild-type (unmutated) KRAS may be candidates for anti-EGFR therapies like cetuximab, while those with mutations may not benefit from these agents.
- **Lung Cancer**: In advanced lung cancer, comprehensive genomic profiling can reveal actionable mutations, such as ALK rearrangements or ROS1 fusions, allowing for the use of targeted therapies like crizotinib or entrectinib, leading to improved outcomes compared to traditional chemotherapy.

4. Challenges and Considerations

While genomic profiling offers promising benefits, several challenges must be addressed:

- **Access and Cost**: The availability and cost of genomic testing can be barriers for some patients. Efforts to improve access and reduce costs are essential for widespread implementation.
- **Interpretation of Results**: Understanding the clinical significance of specific mutations requires expertise. There is a need for ongoing education and resources to support oncologists in interpreting genomic data.
- **Ethical Considerations**: The implications of genetic testing extend beyond immediate treatment decisions, raising ethical questions about privacy, genetic counseling, and potential discrimination.

5. Future Directions in Genomic Profiling

As research advances, the future of genomic profiling in cancer treatment looks promising:

- **Integration with Artificial Intelligence**: The use of AI algorithms to analyze genomic data may enhance the ability to predict treatment responses and identify novel therapeutic targets.
- **Expansion of Testing Panels**: As new mutations and pathways are discovered, expanding genomic testing panels to include more comprehensive gene lists will provide deeper insights into individual tumors.
- **Clinical Trials and Research**: Ongoing clinical trials that explore the impact of genomic profiling on treatment outcomes will be crucial in validating its effectiveness and refining treatment strategies.

Conclusion

Genomic profiling represents a revolutionary approach to personalizing cancer treatment, allowing for more precise and effective therapies tailored to individual patients. By understanding the genetic alterations that drive their cancer, patients can receive targeted treatments that improve outcomes and minimize unnecessary side effects. As the field continues to evolve, integrating genomic profiling into routine clinical practice will be vital in shaping the future of oncology.

In the next chapter, we will explore the collaborative roles of radiologists and oncologists within the multidisciplinary approach to cancer care, emphasizing the importance of teamwork in optimizing patient outcomes and enhancing treatment efficacy.

Chapter 12: Role of Radiologists and Oncologists

Understanding the Multidisciplinary Approach in Oncology, Focusing on Teamwork and Collaboration

The complexity of cancer treatment necessitates a collaborative approach involving a multidisciplinary team of healthcare professionals. Among these, radiologists and oncologists play pivotal roles in diagnosing, planning, and implementing treatment strategies. This chapter explores the distinct and overlapping responsibilities of radiologists and oncologists, emphasizing the importance of teamwork and collaboration in providing optimal patient care.

1. The Role of the Oncologist

Oncologists are physicians who specialize in the diagnosis, treatment, and management of cancer. Their primary responsibilities include:

- **Diagnosis and Staging**: Oncologists use clinical evaluations, imaging studies, and laboratory tests to determine the type and stage of cancer. Accurate staging is crucial for developing an appropriate treatment plan.
- **Treatment Planning**: Based on the diagnosis and staging, oncologists create individualized treatment plans that may include surgery, chemotherapy, radiotherapy, targeted therapy, or immunotherapy. They consider various factors such as tumor characteristics, patient health, and preferences.
- **Patient Management**: Oncologists are responsible for the overall management of cancer patients, monitoring treatment response, managing side effects, and adjusting treatment plans as necessary. They provide ongoing support and guidance throughout the cancer journey.
- **Coordination of Care**: Oncologists act as the central point of contact for patients, coordinating with other specialists, including surgeons, radiologists, pathologists, and palliative care providers to ensure comprehensive care.

2. The Role of the Radiologist

Radiologists are medical doctors specializing in the interpretation of medical imaging and the application of imaging technologies in diagnosing and treating diseases, including cancer. Their key responsibilities include:

- **Diagnostic Imaging**: Radiologists perform and interpret imaging studies such as X-rays, CT scans, MRI scans, and PET scans to identify tumors, assess their extent, and guide treatment planning. Their expertise is critical in the initial diagnosis and ongoing assessment of cancer.
- **Radiation Treatment Planning**: In radiation oncology, radiologists work closely with radiation oncologists to define the target areas for treatment based on imaging studies. They contribute to treatment planning by outlining the anatomy and identifying critical structures to avoid during radiation therapy.
- **Interventional Radiology**: Some radiologists specialize in interventional procedures, which may involve biopsies or the placement of catheters and stents. These procedures can be critical for both diagnosis and treatment, enabling targeted interventions.
- **Follow-Up Imaging**: Radiologists conduct follow-up imaging to assess treatment response, monitor for recurrences, and evaluate any new developments in the patient's condition. They provide essential feedback to oncologists for ongoing management.

3. The Importance of Collaboration

The successful management of cancer patients relies on effective communication and collaboration between radiologists and oncologists. Key aspects of this teamwork include:

- **Case Discussions**: Regular multidisciplinary tumor board meetings allow healthcare professionals to discuss complex cases, share insights, and collaboratively develop comprehensive treatment plans. These discussions ensure that all perspectives are considered, leading to better-informed decisions.
- **Shared Decision-Making**: Collaboration fosters a shared decision-making process, where both the oncologist's treatment expertise and the radiologist's imaging insights are integrated. This approach helps optimize treatment plans based on the latest evidence and the patient's unique circumstances.
- **Integrated Care Pathways**: The establishment of integrated care pathways that outline the roles and responsibilities of each team member enhances continuity of care. Clearly defined protocols ensure that patients receive timely and coordinated treatment.
- **Patient-Centered Approach**: A collaborative approach prioritizes the patient's needs and preferences. By working together, radiologists and oncologists can provide holistic care that addresses not only the disease but also the patient's emotional and psychological well-being.

4. Challenges to Multidisciplinary Collaboration

While collaboration between radiologists and oncologists is essential, several challenges may arise:

- **Communication Barriers**: Effective communication is vital for collaboration. Differences in terminology, reporting formats, and workflows can lead to misunderstandings or delays in patient care.
- **Time Constraints**: The demanding schedules of healthcare professionals can limit opportunities for collaboration. Finding time for discussions and meetings may require deliberate planning and prioritization.
- **Evolving Technologies**: Rapid advancements in imaging and treatment technologies necessitate continuous education and adaptation. Team members must stay informed about new developments to ensure optimal care.

5. Future Directions in Collaborative Oncology Care

As the field of oncology continues to evolve, several trends are shaping the future of collaboration between radiologists and oncologists:

- **Increased Use of Technology**: The integration of advanced imaging technologies, artificial intelligence, and electronic health records can enhance communication and streamline collaborative efforts.
- **Enhanced Training Programs**: Training programs that emphasize multidisciplinary teamwork and communication skills will better prepare future healthcare professionals to work collaboratively in oncology.
- **Research Collaborations**: Collaborative research efforts between radiologists and oncologists will drive innovation and improve treatment strategies, leading to better outcomes for patients.

Conclusion

The roles of radiologists and oncologists are critical in the multidisciplinary approach to cancer care. Effective collaboration between these specialists enhances patient outcomes, facilitates comprehensive treatment planning, and supports a patient-centered approach to care. As the field of oncology continues to advance, fostering strong teamwork and communication will be essential to navigating the complexities of cancer treatment successfully.

In the next chapter, we will discuss the importance of patient assessment and follow-up in oncology, highlighting strategies for monitoring treatment response and ensuring long-term patient well-being. This ongoing evaluation is key to optimizing cancer care and addressing the dynamic needs of patients throughout their treatment journey.

Chapter 13: Patient Assessment and Follow-Up

Importance of Monitoring Treatment Response and Long-Term Follow-Up Strategies

Effective cancer treatment requires ongoing patient assessment and follow-up to evaluate the effectiveness of therapy, manage side effects, and monitor for potential recurrences. This chapter discusses the critical role of patient assessment and follow-up in oncology, including the methodologies employed, key considerations, and the impact on patient outcomes.

1. Objectives of Patient Assessment

Patient assessment serves several key objectives throughout the cancer treatment continuum:

- **Evaluating Treatment Response**: Regular assessments help determine how well a patient is responding to treatment, allowing for timely adjustments to the treatment plan if necessary.
- **Managing Side Effects**: Ongoing monitoring is essential for identifying and managing side effects, ensuring patients maintain their quality of life and adhere to treatment protocols.
- **Detecting Recurrence Early**: Long-term follow-up is crucial for early detection of cancer recurrence, which can significantly improve outcomes if addressed promptly.
- **Assessing Overall Health**: Continuous assessment allows healthcare providers to evaluate a patient's overall health status, which can influence treatment decisions and future care plans.

2. Methods of Patient Assessment

Various methods and tools are employed to assess patients throughout their cancer treatment journey:

a. Clinical Evaluations:

History and Physical Examination

b. Imaging Studies:

Radiologic Assessments

c. Laboratory Tests:

- **Blood Tests**: Routine blood work can help evaluate overall health, monitor organ function, and detect potential issues such as anemia, infection, or abnormalities in tumor markers.
- **Tumor Markers**: Certain cancers produce specific substances in the blood that can indicate treatment response or disease recurrence. Regular monitoring of these markers can guide clinical decisions.

d. Patient-Reported Outcomes (PROs):

Quality of Life Assessments

3. Follow-Up Strategies

Follow-up care is essential for ongoing monitoring and support. Effective follow-up strategies include:

a. Scheduled Appointments:

Establishing a regular follow-up schedule based on the type of cancer and treatment received is critical. This schedule may include frequent visits in the early post-treatment phase, gradually extending the time between visits as appropriate.

b. Survivorship Care Plans:

Developing personalized survivorship care plans that outline the patient's treatment history, follow-up schedule, potential long-term effects, and lifestyle recommendations is essential. These plans empower patients to take an active role in their post-treatment care.

c. Interdisciplinary Coordination:

Collaboration among healthcare providers, including oncologists, primary care physicians, and specialty providers, ensures comprehensive follow-up care. Clear communication among team members is vital to address all aspects of a patient's health.

d. Monitoring for Late Effects:

Some treatments may have delayed side effects that manifest months or years later. Providers should educate patients about potential late effects and ensure regular monitoring for issues such as cardiotoxicity, secondary malignancies, or fertility concerns.

4. Patient Education and Empowerment

Educating patients about the importance of follow-up care and self-monitoring is crucial for improving outcomes. Patients should be informed about:

- **Signs and Symptoms of Recurrence**: Encouraging patients to recognize potential signs of recurrence empowers them to seek timely medical advice.
- **Lifestyle Modifications**: Providing guidance on lifestyle changes, including nutrition, exercise, and smoking cessation, can help support recovery and reduce the risk of recurrence.
- **Psychosocial Support**: Recognizing the emotional challenges of survivorship and connecting patients to support resources can enhance mental well-being.

5. Challenges in Patient Assessment and Follow-Up

Despite the importance of follow-up care, several challenges may arise:

- **Patient Adherence**: Some patients may struggle with regular follow-up visits due to logistical issues, financial constraints, or emotional factors. Healthcare providers must work to address these barriers.
- **Healthcare System Strain**: High patient volumes can limit the time available for comprehensive assessments, impacting the quality of care provided during follow-up appointments.
- **Information Overload**: The complexity of treatment plans and follow-up schedules can be overwhelming for patients. Clear communication and simplified instructions are vital to ensure understanding.

Conclusion

Patient assessment and follow-up are integral components of effective cancer care, contributing to better treatment outcomes and enhanced quality of life. By employing a variety of assessment methods and developing robust follow-up strategies, healthcare providers can monitor treatment response, manage side effects, and detect recurrences early.

In the next chapter, we will discuss the ethical considerations in oncology, exploring the dilemmas faced by healthcare providers and the importance of informed consent and patient autonomy in cancer treatment. Understanding these ethical aspects is essential for delivering compassionate, patient-centered care in oncology.

Chapter 14: Ethical Considerations in Oncology
Discussing the Ethical Dilemmas in Cancer Treatment, Informed Consent, and Patient Autonomy

As cancer treatment evolves, ethical considerations become increasingly significant in guiding the actions and decisions of healthcare providers. Oncologists and multidisciplinary teams face various dilemmas related to patient care, informed consent, and the balancing of risks and benefits. This chapter explores key ethical issues in oncology, emphasizing the importance of patient autonomy, informed decision-making, and equitable access to treatment.

1. Informed Consent

Informed consent is a fundamental ethical principle that ensures patients are fully aware of their treatment options, potential risks, benefits, and consequences. It involves a transparent dialogue between the healthcare provider and the patient.

Key Elements of Informed Consent:

- **Disclosure**: Patients must receive comprehensive information about their diagnosis, proposed treatments, potential side effects, and alternative options. This information should be presented in a way that is understandable and accessible to the patient.
- **Comprehension**: It is vital to ensure that patients understand the information provided. This may involve using visual aids, simplified language, or the assistance of interpreters for patients with language barriers.
- **Voluntariness**: Patients should make decisions without coercion or undue pressure. They must feel free to ask questions and express concerns regarding their treatment options.
- **Competence**: Assessing a patient's capacity to make informed decisions is crucial. Some patients may have cognitive impairments or emotional distress that could impact their ability to fully comprehend the implications of their choices.

Challenges in Informed Consent:

- **Complexity of Information**: The complexities of cancer treatments and the rapid advancements in oncology can make it difficult for patients to grasp all relevant information.
- **Emotional Distress**: The emotional impact of a cancer diagnosis can hinder patients' ability to process information effectively. Healthcare providers must be sensitive to these challenges and provide support throughout the decision-making process.

2. Patient Autonomy

Respecting patient autonomy is a core ethical principle in healthcare. In oncology, this principle emphasizes the right of patients to make informed choices about their treatment, reflecting their values, beliefs, and preferences.

Promoting Patient Autonomy:

- **Shared Decision-Making**: Engaging patients in shared decision-making fosters a collaborative approach. By discussing options and preferences, oncologists can empower patients to take an active role in their care.
- **Advance Care Planning**: Encouraging patients to participate in advance care planning allows them to express their preferences for future medical decisions, particularly regarding end-of-life care.

Ethical Dilemmas:

- **Refusal of Treatment**: Patients may refuse recommended treatments for various reasons, including personal beliefs or concerns about quality of life. Healthcare providers must navigate these situations with empathy while ensuring patients are informed about the potential consequences of their decisions.
- **Informed Consent in Vulnerable Populations**: Special considerations are necessary when obtaining informed consent from vulnerable populations, such as children or patients with cognitive impairments. In these cases, surrogate decision-makers may need to be involved.

3. Balancing Risks and Benefits

Oncologists must often weigh the risks and benefits of various treatment options, which can present ethical challenges:

Risk Assessment:

- **Toxicity vs. Efficacy**: The potential side effects of chemotherapy and radiotherapy can significantly impact a patient's quality of life. Oncologists must carefully assess whether the potential benefits of treatment outweigh the risks, especially in patients with advanced or terminal cancer.
- **Clinical Trials**: The participation of patients in clinical trials raises ethical questions regarding informed consent, the understanding of potential risks, and the balance between experimental treatments and standard care.

4. Equitable Access to Care

Ethical considerations in oncology also encompass issues of access to treatment:

- **Healthcare Disparities**: Disparities in access to cancer care based on socioeconomic status, geographic location, and racial or ethnic backgrounds raise ethical concerns. Efforts to ensure equitable access to advanced therapies and clinical trials are vital for promoting fairness in cancer treatment.
- **Financial Toxicity**: The high costs of cancer treatments can lead to significant financial burdens for patients and their families. Oncologists must be aware of these issues and advocate for patient assistance programs and resources to alleviate financial stress.

5. Future Ethical Considerations

As cancer treatment continues to evolve, new ethical considerations will emerge:

- **Personalized Medicine**: With advancements in genomic profiling and targeted therapies, ethical questions surrounding privacy, genetic discrimination, and informed consent for genetic testing will need to be addressed.
- **Telemedicine**: The increasing use of telemedicine in oncology introduces ethical considerations regarding patient privacy, informed consent, and the quality of care delivered remotely.

Conclusion

Ethical considerations in oncology are multifaceted and vital to ensuring patient-centered care. By prioritizing informed consent, respecting patient autonomy, balancing risks and benefits, and promoting equitable access to care, healthcare providers can navigate the complexities of cancer treatment with integrity and compassion.

In the next chapter, we will explore the psychosocial aspects of cancer treatment, focusing on the emotional and psychological impact of cancer and its treatment on patients and their families. Understanding these factors is essential for providing holistic care that addresses the diverse needs of patients throughout their cancer journey.

Chapter 15: Psychosocial Aspects of Cancer Treatment
Addressing the Emotional and Psychological Impact of Cancer and Its Treatment on Patients and Families

A cancer diagnosis and the subsequent treatment process can profoundly affect a patient's emotional and psychological well-being. Understanding the psychosocial aspects of cancer care is crucial for providing comprehensive treatment that addresses not only the physical aspects of the disease but also the mental and emotional challenges faced by patients and their families. This chapter explores the various psychological impacts of cancer, the importance of supportive care, and strategies to enhance the overall well-being of patients undergoing treatment.

1. Emotional Responses to Cancer Diagnosis

Receiving a cancer diagnosis can trigger a wide range of emotional reactions, including:

- **Shock and Denial**: Many patients experience disbelief or numbness upon receiving their diagnosis, often struggling to accept the reality of their situation.
- **Fear and Anxiety**: Concerns about the cancer's progression, treatment side effects, and the impact on life expectancy can lead to significant anxiety. Patients may also worry about the implications for their loved ones and financial stability.
- **Depression**: Feelings of sadness, hopelessness, and despair can arise as patients confront their diagnosis and treatment challenges. Depression is a common psychological response that can significantly impact treatment adherence and overall quality of life.
- **Anger and Frustration**: Some patients may experience anger towards their diagnosis, healthcare providers, or even themselves. This frustration can stem from feelings of loss of control over their lives.

2. Psychosocial Impact of Treatment

The treatment process itself—whether it involves chemotherapy, radiotherapy, or surgery—can further exacerbate emotional and psychological challenges:

- **Side Effects and Physical Changes**: The physical toll of cancer treatments, such as hair loss, fatigue, and changes in body image, can contribute to feelings of inadequacy and low self-esteem.
- **Isolation and Support Needs**: Cancer treatment can be isolating, as patients may find it challenging to maintain social connections due to fatigue, illness, or the stigma associated with cancer. They may need additional support from family, friends, and healthcare providers.
- **Financial Stress**: The financial burden of cancer treatment can lead to stress and anxiety, impacting mental health. Patients may face high medical costs, loss of income, or challenges accessing adequate insurance coverage.

3. Importance of Supportive Care

Supportive care plays a vital role in addressing the psychosocial aspects of cancer treatment. Key components of supportive care include:

- **Psychological Counseling**: Engaging with mental health professionals, such as psychologists or social workers, can help patients cope with their emotional responses. Counseling can provide patients with tools to manage anxiety, depression, and other psychological challenges.
- **Support Groups**: Participation in support groups allows patients to connect with others facing similar challenges. Sharing experiences and feelings in a supportive environment can reduce feelings of isolation and provide emotional relief.
- **Family Involvement**: Involving family members in the care process can help create a supportive network. Family therapy sessions can also be beneficial in addressing the emotional impact of cancer on family dynamics.
- **Educational Resources**: Providing patients and families with information about the disease, treatment options, and coping strategies can empower them to make informed decisions and alleviate anxiety related to the unknown.

4. Strategies for Enhancing Well-Being

Several strategies can enhance the emotional and psychological well-being of patients undergoing cancer treatment:

- **Mindfulness and Stress Reduction Techniques**: Techniques such as mindfulness meditation, yoga, and relaxation exercises can help patients manage stress and improve overall well-being.
- **Art and Music Therapy**: Engaging in creative activities can provide an outlet for self-expression and emotional processing, helping patients cope with their feelings and reduce anxiety.
- **Physical Activity**: Regular physical activity has been shown to improve mood and reduce anxiety. Encouraging patients to engage in moderate exercise can have positive effects on both mental and physical health.
- **Nutrition and Diet**: A balanced diet can support not only physical health but also mental well-being. Nutritional counseling may help patients make healthier choices that positively impact their mood and energy levels.

5. Addressing Caregiver Stress

The impact of cancer extends beyond patients to their caregivers, who often experience emotional and psychological stress as they support their loved ones. Caregiver stress can manifest as:

- **Emotional Exhaustion**: Caregivers may experience feelings of fatigue, frustration, and helplessness.
- **Impact on Relationships**: The demands of caregiving can strain relationships, leading to conflict and emotional distress.

To address caregiver stress, it is essential to provide support and resources, including respite care options, caregiver support groups, and access to mental health services.

Conclusion

The psychosocial aspects of cancer treatment are critical to ensuring comprehensive care for patients and their families. By addressing the emotional and psychological challenges associated with a cancer diagnosis and its treatment, healthcare providers can enhance patients' quality of life and support their overall well-being. A holistic approach that incorporates supportive care, psychological counseling, and education is essential in navigating the complexities of cancer treatment.

In the next chapter, we will explore the importance of palliative care in oncology, emphasizing symptom management and the role of palliative care in improving quality of life for patients with advanced cancer. Understanding these aspects is crucial for delivering compassionate care throughout the cancer journey.

Chapter 16: Palliative Care in Oncology
Importance of Palliative Care and Symptom Management in Advanced Cancer Cases

Palliative care plays a critical role in the comprehensive treatment of patients with cancer, particularly those with advanced or metastatic disease. This approach prioritizes improving the quality of life by alleviating symptoms, providing psychosocial support, and addressing the complex needs of patients and their families. This chapter explores the principles of palliative care, its benefits, and strategies for effective symptom management in oncology.

1. Understanding Palliative Care

Palliative care is a specialized form of medical care focused on providing relief from the symptoms and stress of serious illness, regardless of the stage of the disease. It aims to enhance the quality of life for both patients and their families through a holistic approach that addresses physical, emotional, spiritual, and social needs.

Key Principles of Palliative Care:

- **Patient-Centered Approach**: Palliative care is tailored to the individual needs of the patient, considering their preferences, values, and cultural background.
- **Interdisciplinary Team**: A multidisciplinary team, including physicians, nurses, social workers, chaplains, and pharmacists, collaborates to provide comprehensive care. Each team member contributes their expertise to address various aspects of the patient's well-being.
- **Early Integration**: Palliative care can be initiated at any point in the disease trajectory, alongside curative or life-prolonging treatments. Early integration into the treatment plan has been shown to improve patient outcomes.

2. Symptom Management

Patients with advanced cancer often experience a variety of distressing symptoms that can significantly impact their quality of life. Effective symptom management is a core component of palliative care.

Common Symptoms and Management Strategies:

Pain Management

- **Pharmacologic Treatments**: Opioids, non-opioid analgesics, and adjuvant medications (e.g., anticonvulsants for neuropathic pain) can be tailored to the patient's needs.
- **Non-Pharmacologic Approaches**: Techniques such as physical therapy, acupuncture, and cognitive-behavioral therapy can complement pharmacological interventions.

Nausea and Vomiting

- **Antiemetic Medications**: Such as ondansetron or metoclopramide, tailored to the underlying cause of nausea.
- **Dietary Modifications**: Encouraging small, frequent meals and avoiding triggers can help manage these symptoms.

Fatigue

- **Activity Management**: Encouraging light physical activity can improve energy levels and reduce fatigue.
- **Addressing Sleep Disturbances**: Sleep hygiene practices and addressing underlying causes of insomnia are essential.

Dyspnea

- **Medications**: Opioids can be effective in reducing the sensation of breathlessness.
- **Oxygen Therapy**: Supplemental oxygen may be beneficial for patients experiencing significant respiratory distress.

Emotional and Psychological Support

- **Psychological Counseling**: Support from mental health professionals can help patients cope with anxiety, depression, and existential distress.
- **Support Groups**: Connecting with peers who share similar experiences can provide emotional support and reduce feelings of isolation.

3. The Role of Palliative Care in the Care Continuum

Palliative care is not limited to end-of-life situations; it plays a vital role throughout the cancer care continuum:

- **Early Intervention**: Initiating palliative care early in the treatment process can enhance symptom management and improve quality of life, even in patients receiving curative treatments.
- **Transition to End-of-Life Care**: As the disease progresses and curative options diminish, palliative care providers can assist with end-of-life planning, advance care directives, and hospice services.
- **Family Support**: Palliative care extends to families, offering support and resources to help them navigate the challenges of caregiving and grief. This holistic approach ensures that both patients and families receive comprehensive care.

4. Overcoming Barriers to Palliative Care

Despite its benefits, several barriers to accessing palliative care may exist:

- **Misconceptions**: There is often a misunderstanding that palliative care is synonymous with end-of-life care. Educating patients, families, and healthcare providers about the scope of palliative care is essential.
- **Access to Services**: Availability of palliative care services can vary by region, with some areas lacking adequate resources. Advocacy for the expansion of palliative care programs is vital to improve access for all patients.
- **Integration into Oncology**: Integrating palliative care into standard oncology practices can be challenging. Training oncologists and healthcare teams in palliative care principles can facilitate this integration.

Conclusion

Palliative care is an essential component of cancer treatment, focusing on improving the quality of life for patients and their families. By addressing symptoms, providing emotional support, and facilitating communication, palliative care enhances the overall cancer care experience. As the field of oncology continues to evolve, the integration of palliative care alongside curative and life-prolonging treatments will play a crucial role in delivering compassionate, patient-centered care.

In the next chapter, we will explore the role of nutrition in cancer treatment, examining how dietary choices can support patients undergoing radiotherapy and chemotherapy. Understanding the importance of nutrition is vital for optimizing patient health and well-being throughout the treatment journey.

Chapter 17: Nutrition and Cancer Treatment

Exploring the Role of Nutrition in Supporting Patients Undergoing Radiotherapy and Chemotherapy

Nutrition plays a vital role in the overall health and well-being of cancer patients. It can significantly impact treatment outcomes, support recovery, and enhance the quality of life during and after treatment. This chapter delves into the importance of nutrition in oncology, discussing dietary recommendations, the management of treatment-related side effects, and the role of nutrition in survivorship.

1. The Importance of Nutrition in Cancer Care

Proper nutrition is crucial for cancer patients for several reasons:

- **Maintaining Nutritional Status**: Cancer and its treatments can lead to malnutrition, weight loss, and muscle wasting. Adequate nutrition helps maintain a healthy weight and preserves lean body mass, which is essential for recovery and overall health.
- **Supporting Immune Function**: A well-balanced diet can enhance the immune system, helping patients better tolerate treatments and reducing the risk of infections during periods of immunosuppression.
- **Managing Treatment Side Effects**: Good nutrition can help mitigate some side effects of cancer treatments, such as nausea, vomiting, fatigue, and loss of appetite. Specific dietary strategies can alleviate discomfort and promote better adherence to treatment regimens.
- **Enhancing Treatment Efficacy**: Emerging evidence suggests that certain nutrients may enhance the effectiveness of cancer therapies. For instance, antioxidants can protect healthy cells from oxidative stress caused by radiation therapy.

2. Nutritional Recommendations During Treatment

Dietary recommendations for cancer patients should be individualized based on their treatment type, side effects, and nutritional needs. However, several general guidelines can be beneficial:

a. Balanced Diet:

Encourage a variety of foods from all food groups, including fruits, vegetables, whole grains, lean proteins, and healthy fats. This approach ensures an adequate intake of essential nutrients, vitamins, and minerals.

b. Hydration:

Maintaining hydration is crucial, particularly for patients experiencing vomiting or diarrhea due to treatment. Encourage the intake of fluids, including water, herbal teas, and broths.

c. High-Calorie, High-Protein Foods:

Patients undergoing treatment may require additional calories and protein to support healing and energy levels. Suggestions include:

- Whole milk, cheese, yogurt, and smoothies.
- Nut butters, seeds, and avocados for healthy fats.
- Protein-rich foods such as eggs, beans, lentils, and lean meats.

d. Small, Frequent Meals:

Eating small, frequent meals can help manage nausea and improve appetite. Patients should be encouraged to eat what they feel comfortable with, even if it's not a traditional meal.

3. Managing Specific Side Effects Through Nutrition

Cancer treatments can cause various side effects that affect nutritional intake. Understanding how to manage these side effects through dietary strategies is essential:

a. Nausea and Vomiting:

- **Ginger**: Incorporating ginger tea or ginger ale can help alleviate nausea.
- **Bland Foods**: Recommend bland, low-fat foods such as crackers, toast, and bananas.
- **Avoiding Triggers**: Patients should identify and avoid foods that exacerbate nausea.

b. Taste Changes:

- **Experiment with Flavors**: Patients may experience changes in taste; encourage them to experiment with different seasonings and flavors to enhance the palatability of meals.
- **Cold Foods**: Cold or room-temperature foods may be more appealing than hot meals.

c. Mouth Sores and Mucositis:

- **Soft Foods**: Suggest soft, non-irritating foods such as mashed potatoes, smoothies, and oatmeal.
- **Oral Care**: Encourage good oral hygiene and the use of mouth rinses to soothe irritation.

d. Diarrhea:

- **Bland Diet**: Foods such as bananas, rice, applesauce, and toast (the BRAT diet) can help manage diarrhea.
- **Probiotics**: Incorporating probiotics, such as yogurt or supplements, may help restore gut health.

4. Nutritional Considerations After Treatment

Post-treatment nutrition is equally important for recovery and survivorship:

- **Focus on Whole Foods**: Encourage a diet rich in whole, minimally processed foods to support overall health and reduce the risk of recurrence.
- **Weight Management**: Help patients achieve and maintain a healthy weight through balanced nutrition and regular physical activity.
- **Regular Follow-Up**: Continued nutritional assessment and support may be necessary, particularly for those experiencing long-term side effects from treatment.

5. Collaborating with Nutrition Professionals

Integrating the expertise of registered dietitians or nutritionists into the cancer care team can enhance nutritional management. These professionals can provide personalized dietary recommendations, create meal plans, and address specific nutritional concerns related to cancer treatment.

Conclusion

Nutrition is a critical component of cancer care that can significantly influence treatment outcomes and quality of life for patients undergoing radiotherapy and chemotherapy. By understanding the role of nutrition, implementing tailored dietary strategies, and providing ongoing support, healthcare providers can empower patients to optimize their health and well-being throughout their cancer journey.

In the next chapter, we will explore clinical trials and research advances, highlighting their importance in developing new treatments and improving existing ones. Understanding the role of clinical research is essential for enhancing cancer care and advancing the field of oncology.

Chapter 18: Clinical Trials and Research Advances

Overview of Ongoing Clinical Trials and Their Importance in Advancing Cancer Treatment

Clinical trials are critical for advancing our understanding of cancer and improving treatment modalities. They provide a structured approach to testing new therapies, drugs, and techniques, ultimately leading to innovations in cancer care. This chapter discusses the purpose and phases of clinical trials, the role they play in oncology, and how patients can engage with this vital aspect of cancer treatment.

1. Understanding Clinical Trials

Clinical trials are research studies that test the effectiveness and safety of new interventions in human participants. These interventions may include new drugs, surgical techniques, radiation therapies, or combinations of treatments. The primary objectives of clinical trials are to evaluate:

- **Efficacy**: How well a new treatment works in comparison to standard therapies.
- **Safety**: Assessing any adverse effects or potential risks associated with a new treatment.
- **Dosage**: Determining the appropriate dose of a drug that maximizes effectiveness while minimizing side effects.

2. Phases of Clinical Trials

Clinical trials are conducted in distinct phases, each designed to answer specific research questions:

Phase 1:

- **Objective**: Evaluate the safety and tolerability of a new treatment in a small group of participants (typically 20-100).
- **Focus**: Determine the maximum tolerated dose and identify side effects.
- **Participants**: Often include patients with advanced cancer who have exhausted other treatment options.

Phase 2:

- **Objective**: Assess the effectiveness of the treatment while continuing to evaluate its safety.
- **Focus**: Determine the treatment's efficacy in a larger group (typically 100-300) of patients with a specific type of cancer.
- **Outcome Measures**: Effectiveness is often measured by tumor response rates or progression-free survival.

Phase 3:

- **Objective**: Compare the new treatment to the current standard of care in a larger patient population (typically several hundred to several thousand).
- **Focus**: Confirm the treatment's effectiveness, monitor side effects, and collect information that will allow the treatment to be used safely.
- **Randomization**: Participants are often randomly assigned to receive either the new treatment or the standard treatment to ensure unbiased results.

Phase 4:

- **Objective**: Conducted after a treatment has been approved by regulatory agencies to gather additional information on its risks, benefits, and optimal use.
- **Focus**: Long-term effectiveness and safety data are collected to monitor any rare or long-term side effects.

3. The Role of Clinical Trials in Oncology

Clinical trials play an essential role in cancer treatment and research for several reasons:

- **Innovation**: They facilitate the development of new therapies and treatment strategies that can lead to breakthroughs in cancer care.
- **Evidence-Based Practice**: Results from clinical trials provide the evidence needed to inform clinical practice and guidelines, helping oncologists make better treatment decisions.
- **Personalized Medicine**: Trials increasingly focus on targeted therapies and personalized approaches, improving treatment outcomes by matching patients with the most effective therapies based on their genetic profiles.
- **Quality of Life Improvements**: Many trials assess not only survival rates but also the impact of treatments on patients' quality of life, ensuring that the benefits of new therapies outweigh their risks.

4. Patient Participation in Clinical Trials

Participating in clinical trials can offer patients access to cutting-edge treatments and contribute to advancements in cancer care. Key considerations for patients include:

- **Informed Consent**: Patients must be thoroughly informed about the trial's purpose, procedures, risks, and benefits before consenting to participate. This ensures that they make an educated decision about their involvement.
- **Eligibility Criteria**: Each trial has specific inclusion and exclusion criteria based on factors such as cancer type, stage, previous treatments, and overall health. Patients should discuss with their healthcare team whether they qualify for any ongoing trials.
- **Potential Risks and Benefits**: Patients should weigh the potential risks and benefits of participation. While some may receive access to promising new therapies, others may experience side effects or receive a placebo.
- **Support Systems**: Family members and caregivers should be involved in discussions about clinical trials, as they can provide support and help patients navigate the decision-making process.

5. Finding Clinical Trials

Several resources are available for patients seeking clinical trial opportunities:

- **ClinicalTrials.gov**: A comprehensive database of publicly and privately funded clinical trials conducted worldwide, allowing patients to search by location, condition, and treatment.
- **Cancer Centers and Research Institutions**: Many cancer treatment centers have ongoing clinical trials and can provide information about participation options.
- **Oncology Specialists**: Healthcare providers can offer guidance and recommendations regarding suitable trials based on the patient's specific cancer diagnosis and treatment history.

Conclusion

Clinical trials are fundamental to advancing cancer treatment and improving patient outcomes. They provide a pathway for innovation, enhance the understanding of cancer therapies, and enable personalized medicine approaches. Encouraging patient participation and ensuring informed decision-making are essential components of this process.

In the next chapter, we will explore the importance of safety and quality assurance in radiotherapy, discussing protocols and measures in place to ensure patient safety and treatment efficacy in radiation oncology. Understanding these safety measures is crucial for delivering high-quality cancer care.

Chapter 19: Radiotherapy Safety and Quality Assurance

Ensuring Safety Protocols and Quality Assurance Measures in Radiation Oncology

Radiotherapy is a cornerstone of cancer treatment, providing targeted doses of radiation to eradicate malignant cells while minimizing exposure to healthy tissues. Given the potential risks associated with radiation exposure, ensuring patient safety and implementing robust quality assurance measures are paramount. This chapter discusses the critical safety protocols and quality assurance practices in radiation oncology, aiming to enhance patient outcomes and mitigate risks.

1. Understanding Radiotherapy Safety

Radiotherapy safety encompasses various practices designed to protect patients from unnecessary exposure to radiation and ensure the accurate delivery of treatment. The following key principles guide safety in radiotherapy:

- **Justification**: Every radiotherapy treatment must be justified, meaning the expected benefits of treatment should outweigh the potential risks associated with radiation exposure. This principle underscores the importance of thorough patient evaluation and consideration of alternative therapies.
- **Optimization**: Once a treatment is justified, optimization involves using the lowest radiation dose necessary to achieve the desired therapeutic effect. Techniques such as image-guided radiotherapy (IGRT) allow for precise targeting of tumors, enhancing treatment efficacy while protecting surrounding healthy tissue.
- **Adherence to Protocols**: Strict adherence to clinical protocols and guidelines is essential for maintaining safety. These protocols outline the steps involved in patient treatment, from initial planning to treatment delivery and follow-up.

2. Key Safety Protocols in Radiotherapy

Safety protocols are integral to ensuring the protection of patients and staff in radiation oncology settings. Important safety measures include:

a. Equipment Quality Assurance:

Regular maintenance and calibration of radiation delivery equipment (linear accelerators, brachytherapy devices) are vital for ensuring accurate dose delivery. Quality assurance tests should be conducted according to established standards and regulatory guidelines.

b. Treatment Planning Verification:

Treatment plans must undergo thorough verification processes before implementation. This includes independent double-checks by qualified personnel to confirm that the calculated doses and treatment parameters align with the prescribed plan.

c. Patient Identification and Verification:

Ensuring that the correct patient receives the correct treatment is paramount. Protocols must be in place for verifying patient identity, treatment site, and treatment plan before each session, commonly referred to as "time out" procedures.

d. Safety Training:

Continuous education and training for healthcare professionals involved in radiotherapy are essential. Staff should be well-versed in safety protocols, emergency procedures, and the latest advancements in radiation technology.

3. Quality Assurance Measures in Radiotherapy

Quality assurance (QA) is a systematic process aimed at maintaining and improving the quality of radiotherapy delivery. Key QA measures include:

a. Regular Audits and Inspections:

Periodic audits of radiation oncology practices help identify areas for improvement and ensure compliance with safety standards. Inspections by regulatory bodies also play a role in maintaining high-quality care.

b. Incident Reporting and Analysis:

Establishing a culture of safety involves encouraging the reporting of any incidents or near misses related to radiation treatment. Analyzing these events can help identify root causes and implement corrective actions to prevent recurrence.

c. Patient Follow-Up and Feedback:

Monitoring patient outcomes after radiotherapy treatment is crucial for quality assurance. Collecting patient feedback regarding their experiences can provide insights into areas that may require enhancement.

d. Integration of Technology:

Advancements in technology, such as electronic health records and computerized treatment planning systems, can enhance quality assurance efforts by improving data accuracy, reducing human error, and streamlining communication among the care team.

4. Patient Education and Involvement

Patient safety in radiotherapy also involves educating patients about their treatment. Effective communication fosters an understanding of the treatment process, potential side effects, and safety measures:

- **Informed Consent**: Patients should receive comprehensive information about the risks and benefits of radiotherapy, including safety protocols. This enables them to make informed decisions about their treatment.
- **Engagement in Safety Practices**: Patients can play a role in their safety by actively participating in verification processes, asking questions, and reporting any concerns during treatment.

5. Future Directions in Radiotherapy Safety and Quality Assurance

As technology continues to evolve, several trends are shaping the future of safety and quality assurance in radiotherapy:

- **Artificial Intelligence (AI)**: AI can assist in treatment planning, patient monitoring, and quality assurance processes by identifying discrepancies and optimizing treatment parameters, enhancing both safety and efficacy.
- **Patient-Centered Approaches**: Emphasizing patient involvement in safety practices and decision-making can improve treatment experiences and outcomes, leading to a more holistic approach to care.
- **Research and Innovation**: Ongoing research into novel radiation techniques, such as stereotactic body radiotherapy (SBRT) and proton therapy, will require the continuous development of safety protocols and quality assurance measures specific to these modalities.

Conclusion

Ensuring safety and quality assurance in radiotherapy is paramount to providing effective cancer treatment while minimizing risks to patients. By adhering to established safety protocols, implementing robust quality assurance measures, and engaging patients in their care, healthcare professionals can enhance the overall safety of radiation oncology practices.

In the next chapter, we will discuss best practices for administering chemotherapy and monitoring for complications. Understanding these practices is crucial for optimizing patient outcomes and managing the complexities of cancer treatment.

Chapter 20: Chemotherapy Administration and Monitoring

Best Practices for Administering Chemotherapy and Monitoring for Complications

Chemotherapy remains a cornerstone in the treatment of various cancers, utilizing potent drugs to target and kill cancer cells. However, its administration comes with significant responsibilities regarding patient safety and monitoring for adverse effects. This chapter outlines best practices for chemotherapy administration, effective monitoring strategies, and the management of complications that may arise during treatment.

1. Preparing for Chemotherapy Administration

Effective chemotherapy administration begins with thorough preparation and planning:

a. Patient Assessment:

- **Comprehensive Evaluation**: Before chemotherapy initiation, healthcare providers should conduct a detailed assessment of the patient's medical history, including previous treatments, comorbidities, and current medications. This assessment aids in tailoring the chemotherapy regimen to the individual patient's needs.
- **Laboratory Tests**: Blood tests should be performed to evaluate organ function (liver and kidney), blood counts (CBC), and any relevant tumor markers. These tests help determine the patient's eligibility for treatment and guide dosing decisions.

b. Education and Informed Consent:

- **Patient Education**: Inform patients about the chemotherapy drugs, expected side effects, treatment schedule, and what to expect during administration. This education empowers patients and helps alleviate anxiety.
- **Informed Consent**: Obtain informed consent by ensuring that patients understand the risks and benefits of chemotherapy, as well as any alternatives available.

c. Setting Up the Environment:

Designated Chemotherapy Area

2. Administration of Chemotherapy

Chemotherapy can be administered through various routes, including intravenous (IV), oral, intramuscular (IM), or subcutaneous (SC). Each method has its protocols and best practices:

a. Intravenous Administration:

- **Venous Access**: Use appropriate venous access devices, such as peripheral IV lines or central venous catheters, to ensure safe delivery of chemotherapy. The choice of access device should be based on the expected duration and frequency of treatment.
- **Infusion Protocols**: Follow standardized infusion protocols, including premedication if indicated (e.g., for antiemetics) and the rate of infusion. Monitor the patient closely during infusion for signs of adverse reactions.

b. Oral Chemotherapy:

- **Patient Education**: Ensure patients understand how to take oral chemotherapy correctly, including dosing schedules and the importance of adherence. Discuss potential side effects and when to seek medical advice.
- **Monitoring for Toxicity**: Regularly assess the patient's ability to tolerate the medication, including monitoring for gastrointestinal side effects and blood counts.

3. Monitoring for Complications

Monitoring patients during and after chemotherapy administration is critical for identifying and managing complications:

a. Immediate Monitoring:

- **Vital Signs**: Continuously monitor vital signs during infusion, including blood pressure, heart rate, respiratory rate, and temperature, to identify any acute reactions.
- **Assessment of Infusion Site**: Check for signs of infiltration, extravasation, or phlebitis at the infusion site. Any abnormalities should be addressed immediately to prevent tissue damage.

b. Early Detection of Side Effects:

- **Adverse Reactions**: Be vigilant for immediate and delayed adverse reactions, such as allergic reactions, fever, nausea, vomiting, or changes in blood counts. Establish a clear protocol for managing these events.
- **Patient Communication**: Encourage patients to report any unusual symptoms promptly, ensuring they feel supported and aware of the importance of communication.

c. Long-Term Monitoring:

- **Follow-Up Visits**: Schedule regular follow-up appointments to monitor for late-onset side effects, such as cardiotoxicity, neurotoxicity, or secondary malignancies.
- **Laboratory Monitoring**: Periodically assess blood counts and organ function tests throughout the treatment course to detect potential toxicities early and adjust treatment plans as necessary.

4. Managing Complications

Effective management of complications is essential to ensure patient safety and treatment continuity:

a. Nausea and Vomiting:

Proactive Management

b. Neutropenia:

Monitoring and Intervention

c. Anemia and Thrombocytopenia:

Supportive Care

5. Patient Support and Resources

Supportive care is crucial in helping patients cope with the physical and emotional challenges of chemotherapy:

- **Psychosocial Support**: Provide access to counseling services, support groups, and educational resources to help patients navigate the emotional impact of cancer treatment.
- **Nutritional Support**: Collaborate with dietitians to ensure patients receive adequate nutrition to support recovery and manage treatment-related side effects.

Conclusion

The administration of chemotherapy and the monitoring for complications are integral components of cancer treatment. By adhering to best practices for safe administration, vigilant monitoring, and effective management of side effects, healthcare providers can optimize patient outcomes and enhance the quality of life for individuals undergoing chemotherapy.

In the next chapter, we will explore future directions in cancer treatment, focusing on emerging trends, technologies, and therapies that are shaping the landscape of oncology. Understanding these advancements is crucial for adapting to the ever-evolving field of cancer care.

Chapter 21: Future Directions in Cancer Treatment

Insights into Emerging Trends, Technologies, and Therapies Shaping the Future of Oncology

The landscape of cancer treatment is continuously evolving, driven by research, technological advancements, and a deeper understanding of cancer biology. As we look to the future, several key trends and innovations are poised to shape the direction of oncology, enhancing the efficacy and safety of cancer treatments. This chapter explores the future directions in cancer treatment, focusing on personalized medicine, innovative therapies, technology integration, and the importance of holistic approaches.

1. Personalized Medicine

Personalized medicine, or precision oncology, aims to tailor treatments based on individual patient characteristics, including genetics, tumor biology, and lifestyle factors. This approach is becoming increasingly prominent in cancer care, with several developments:

- **Genomic Profiling**: The integration of genomic profiling into clinical practice allows for the identification of specific mutations and biomarkers associated with various cancers. Targeted therapies can be developed based on these profiles, leading to more effective and individualized treatment plans.
- **Liquid Biopsies**: Liquid biopsies, which analyze circulating tumor DNA (ctDNA) from blood samples, offer a non-invasive method for monitoring tumor dynamics, treatment response, and potential resistance mechanisms. This technology holds promise for early detection and real-time assessment of treatment efficacy.
- **Biomarker-Driven Therapies**: As the understanding of tumor biology expands, the development of biomarker-driven therapies will enable oncologists to select the most effective treatments for individual patients. This approach enhances treatment outcomes and minimizes unnecessary toxicity.

2. Innovative Therapies

The future of cancer treatment is marked by the emergence of several innovative therapies that go beyond traditional chemotherapy and radiotherapy:

- **Immunotherapy**: Immunotherapy has revolutionized cancer treatment by harnessing the body's immune system to target and destroy cancer cells. Advances in monoclonal antibodies, checkpoint inhibitors, and CAR T-cell therapies have shown remarkable efficacy in various cancers. Ongoing research continues to explore combination strategies to enhance responses and overcome resistance.
- **Targeted Therapies**: Targeted therapies focus on specific molecular targets involved in cancer progression. The development of new targeted agents continues to expand, with ongoing trials exploring combinations of targeted therapies and immunotherapies to improve patient outcomes.
- **Oncolytic Virus Therapy**: Oncolytic virus therapy involves using genetically modified viruses that selectively infect and kill cancer cells while sparing healthy tissue. This approach is being investigated in various cancers and offers a novel treatment modality with the potential for enhanced efficacy.
- **Gene Therapy**: Gene therapy techniques, such as CRISPR/Cas9 technology, are being explored to correct genetic mutations or modify the expression of genes involved in cancer. These innovative approaches hold promise for personalized treatment strategies.

3. Integration of Technology

Technological advancements are transforming the field of oncology, improving both treatment delivery and patient monitoring:

- **Artificial Intelligence (AI)**: AI and machine learning algorithms are increasingly being used to analyze complex datasets, aiding in treatment decision-making, predicting outcomes, and identifying patterns in patient responses. AI tools can enhance the accuracy of diagnostics and treatment planning.
- **Telemedicine**: The use of telemedicine has surged, providing patients with convenient access to care and follow-up consultations. This approach improves patient engagement and adherence to treatment plans, particularly for those in remote areas or with mobility challenges.
- **Wearable Technology**: Wearable devices that monitor vital signs, physical activity, and symptoms can provide real-time data on patient health. This information allows healthcare providers to tailor interventions and support based on individual patient needs.

4. Holistic and Integrative Approaches

The future of cancer treatment recognizes the importance of a holistic approach to patient care:

- **Mind-Body Interventions**: Techniques such as mindfulness, yoga, and meditation are gaining recognition for their role in enhancing patients' emotional and psychological well-being. Integrating these practices into standard oncology care can improve patients' quality of life.
- **Nutritional Support**: Ongoing research highlights the impact of nutrition on treatment outcomes and survivorship. Tailoring dietary interventions to support patients throughout their treatment journey is becoming increasingly important.
- **Patient-Centered Care**: Emphasizing patient-centered care, where patients actively participate in their treatment decisions and care plans, is essential for improving satisfaction and outcomes. This approach fosters a collaborative relationship between patients and healthcare providers.

5. Research and Collaboration

Collaboration among researchers, healthcare providers, and patients is crucial for advancing cancer treatment:

- **Interdisciplinary Research**: Collaborative efforts across disciplines, including oncology, genomics, immunology, and bioinformatics, will drive innovation and accelerate the development of new therapies.
- **Patient Involvement in Research**: Engaging patients in research initiatives, such as patient-reported outcomes and involvement in clinical trial design, can provide valuable insights that enhance the relevance and applicability of research findings.

Conclusion

The future of cancer treatment is characterized by personalized approaches, innovative therapies, and the integration of advanced technologies. As we continue to deepen our understanding of cancer biology and harness the power of precision medicine, the potential for improved outcomes and enhanced quality of life for patients is substantial.

In the next chapter, we will explore patient education and support resources, emphasizing the importance of empowering patients with knowledge and tools to navigate their cancer treatment journey effectively. Understanding these resources is essential for fostering patient engagement and improving overall care.

Chapter 22: Patient Education and Support Resources

Strategies for Educating Patients and Providing Resources for Support During Treatment

Effective patient education and support are vital components of cancer care, significantly influencing treatment adherence, patient satisfaction, and overall health outcomes. This chapter discusses the strategies for educating patients about their treatment options and the resources available to support them throughout their cancer journey.

1. Importance of Patient Education

Patient education empowers individuals to understand their condition, treatment options, and potential side effects. Key benefits of effective patient education include:

- **Informed Decision-Making**: Educated patients can make informed choices regarding their treatment plans, which can enhance their engagement and satisfaction with care.
- **Improved Adherence**: When patients understand the rationale behind their treatment and the importance of adherence, they are more likely to follow through with prescribed regimens.
- **Enhanced Self-Management**: Knowledge equips patients to manage symptoms, recognize side effects, and take proactive steps in their care, ultimately improving their quality of life.

2. Effective Education Strategies

To maximize the effectiveness of patient education, healthcare providers should consider the following strategies:

a. Tailored Information:

Individualized Education

b. Use of Clear Language:

Simplified Terminology

c. Visual Aids:

Educational Materials

d. Active Engagement:

Encourage Questions

e. Teach-Back Method:

Assessment of Understanding

3. Providing Comprehensive Resources

In addition to direct education, healthcare providers should ensure that patients have access to various support resources:

a. Support Groups:

Peer Support

b. Counseling Services:

Emotional Support

c. Nutritional Counseling:

Dietary Guidance

d. Educational Workshops:

Informative Sessions

e. Online Resources:

Access to Information

4. Involving Families and Caregivers

Involving family members and caregivers in the educational process is crucial, as they play a significant role in supporting patients throughout their treatment:

- **Family Education**: Provide education for family members about the patient's diagnosis, treatment plan, and potential side effects. This knowledge equips them to offer informed support.
- **Encouragement of Involvement**: Encourage family participation during medical appointments. Having loved ones present can help patients remember information and provide emotional support.

5. Leveraging Technology for Education and Support

Technology can enhance patient education and support through various platforms:

a. Telehealth Services:

Remote Education

b. Mobile Applications:

Health Tracking

c. Online Patient Portals:

Access to Information

Conclusion

Effective patient education and support resources are essential components of comprehensive cancer care. By employing tailored education strategies, providing access to resources, and involving families, healthcare providers can empower patients to actively participate in their treatment journey. This empowerment not only enhances adherence and satisfaction but also contributes to improved health outcomes and quality of life.

In the next chapter, we will explore integrative approaches in cancer care, examining how complementary therapies can be used in conjunction with conventional treatments to support patients holistically throughout their cancer journey. Understanding these integrative approaches is crucial for fostering comprehensive care in oncology.

Chapter 23: Integrative Approaches in Cancer Care
Exploring Complementary Therapies and Their Role in Conjunction with Conventional Treatments

The landscape of cancer care is increasingly recognizing the importance of integrative approaches that combine conventional treatments, such as chemotherapy and radiotherapy, with complementary therapies. This chapter discusses various integrative strategies, their benefits, and how they can enhance patient outcomes, support symptom management, and improve overall well-being during the cancer treatment journey.

1. Understanding Integrative Cancer Care

Integrative cancer care involves the coordination of conventional medical treatments with complementary therapies to address the physical, emotional, and psychological needs of patients. This holistic approach emphasizes treating the patient as a whole rather than focusing solely on the disease.

Key Components:

- **Holistic Approach**: Integrative care considers all aspects of a patient's health, including physical, emotional, social, and spiritual well-being.
- **Patient-Centered Care**: Emphasizes active participation of patients in their treatment plans, allowing them to choose therapies that align with their values and preferences.
- **Collaboration among Providers**: Encourages collaboration between oncologists, complementary therapy practitioners, and other healthcare providers to create comprehensive treatment plans.

2. Common Complementary Therapies

A variety of complementary therapies can be integrated into cancer care, each offering unique benefits:

a. Mind-Body Techniques:

- **Mindfulness and Meditation**: Practices that promote relaxation, reduce stress, and enhance emotional resilience. Mindfulness-based interventions can improve coping strategies and quality of life for cancer patients.
- **Yoga and Tai Chi**: These physical activities promote relaxation, enhance physical fitness, and reduce fatigue and anxiety. They can be tailored to accommodate individual patient needs and abilities.

b. Nutritional Therapy:

- **Dietary Interventions**: Nutrition plays a vital role in supporting cancer patients. Dietitians can provide personalized dietary plans that promote healing, manage side effects, and optimize nutritional intake during treatment.
- **Supplements**: Some patients may benefit from specific supplements, such as vitamins, minerals, and herbal products. However, these should always be discussed with healthcare providers to avoid interactions with conventional treatments.

c. Acupuncture:

Pain and Symptom Management

d. Massage and Bodywork:

Stress Relief and Relaxation

e. Music and Art Therapy:

Emotional Expression

3. Benefits of Integrative Approaches

Integrative approaches can offer several benefits to cancer patients:

- **Enhanced Quality of Life**: Complementary therapies can improve physical, emotional, and social well-being, leading to an overall better quality of life during treatment.
- **Symptom Management**: Integrative therapies can help manage common symptoms associated with cancer and its treatments, such as pain, fatigue, nausea, and anxiety.
- **Improved Treatment Tolerance**: Patients who engage in integrative therapies often report a better ability to tolerate conventional treatments, leading to improved adherence to treatment plans.
- **Empowerment**: Involving patients in their care through complementary therapies fosters a sense of empowerment and control over their health journey.

4. Considerations for Integrative Care

While integrative approaches can provide significant benefits, there are essential considerations to ensure their safe and effective implementation:

- **Communication with Healthcare Providers**: Patients should discuss their interest in complementary therapies with their healthcare team to ensure coordination and avoid potential interactions with conventional treatments.
- **Evidence-Based Practices**: Healthcare providers should focus on therapies supported by scientific evidence, ensuring that patients receive safe and effective interventions.
- **Individualized Treatment Plans**: Complementary therapies should be tailored to the unique needs of each patient, considering their preferences, treatment stage, and overall health status.

5. Research and Future Directions

Ongoing research into integrative therapies is vital for understanding their effectiveness and establishing best practices. Future directions may include:

- **Clinical Trials**: Investigating the efficacy of specific complementary therapies in conjunction with conventional treatments through well-designed clinical trials.
- **Standardization of Practices**: Developing standardized protocols for integrating complementary therapies into cancer care to enhance consistency and safety.
- **Education and Training**: Increasing education and training for healthcare providers in integrative oncology practices to promote collaboration and enhance patient care.

Conclusion

Integrative approaches in cancer care represent a promising frontier that enhances the treatment experience for patients. By combining conventional treatments with complementary therapies, healthcare providers can address the diverse needs of patients, promoting their physical, emotional, and psychological well-being. As the field of oncology continues to evolve, integrating these approaches will play a crucial role in delivering comprehensive, patient-centered care.

In the next chapter, we will examine real-life case studies in radiotherapy and chemotherapy, highlighting treatment decisions and outcomes that illustrate the principles discussed throughout the book. Understanding these cases will provide valuable insights into practical applications of the knowledge acquired in mastering cancer care.

Chapter 24: Case Studies in Radiotherapy and Chemotherapy

Real-Life Case Studies Highlighting Treatment Decisions and Outcomes

Case studies provide valuable insights into the practical application of theoretical knowledge in oncology. By examining real-life scenarios, healthcare professionals can learn from the experiences of others, recognize challenges, and identify effective strategies in managing cancer treatment. This chapter presents a series of case studies that illustrate key concepts in radiotherapy and chemotherapy, focusing on treatment decisions, patient outcomes, and the lessons learned.

Case Study 1: Advanced Non-Small Cell Lung Cancer (NSCLC)

Patient Profile:

- **Age:** 67
- **Gender:** Male
- **Diagnosis:** Stage IIIB Non-Small Cell Lung Cancer

Treatment Plan: The patient presented with a primary tumor in the right lung and multiple lymph node metastases. After a thorough evaluation, the oncology team decided on a combination of chemotherapy and radiation therapy. The treatment plan included:

1. **Chemotherapy:** The patient was started on a regimen of cisplatin and pemetrexed, administered every three weeks.
2. **Radiotherapy:** Concurrently, the patient received daily radiation therapy using intensity-modulated radiotherapy (IMRT) to minimize exposure to surrounding healthy tissues.

Outcomes:

- The patient tolerated the chemotherapy regimen well with manageable side effects, primarily mild nausea and fatigue.
- After six cycles of chemotherapy and 30 sessions of radiation, imaging showed a significant reduction in tumor size and lymph node involvement.

Lessons Learned:

- The use of concurrent chemoradiotherapy was effective in enhancing treatment outcomes in this patient with advanced lung cancer.
- Regular monitoring of side effects allowed for timely interventions, ensuring adherence to the treatment protocol.

Case Study 2: Breast Cancer with Neoadjuvant Therapy

Patient Profile:

- **Age**: 52
- **Gender**: Female
- **Diagnosis**: Stage II Estrogen Receptor-Positive Breast Cancer

Treatment Plan: The patient was diagnosed with a 3 cm tumor in the left breast. A multidisciplinary team recommended neoadjuvant chemotherapy followed by surgery to reduce tumor size before surgical intervention. The treatment plan included:

1. **Neoadjuvant Chemotherapy**: The patient received four cycles of doxorubicin and cyclophosphamide, followed by four cycles of paclitaxel.
2. **Surgery**: After chemotherapy, the patient underwent a lumpectomy with sentinel lymph node biopsy.
3. **Adjuvant Radiotherapy**: Post-surgery, the patient received 30 fractions of adjuvant radiotherapy to the left breast.

Outcomes:

- Imaging after neoadjuvant therapy revealed a significant decrease in tumor size, allowing for a successful lumpectomy.
- Post-surgical pathology showed no lymph node involvement and a clear margin.

Lessons Learned:

- Neoadjuvant chemotherapy provided the benefit of tumor shrinkage, enabling breast-conserving surgery and optimizing surgical outcomes.
- Collaboration among surgical, medical, and radiation oncologists was crucial for ensuring comprehensive care.

Case Study 3: Pediatric Hodgkin Lymphoma

Patient Profile:

- **Age**: 14
- **Gender**: Female
- **Diagnosis**: Stage IIB Hodgkin Lymphoma

Treatment Plan: The patient was diagnosed after presenting with cervical lymphadenopathy and fever. A treatment plan was developed as follows:

1. **Chemotherapy**: The patient received ABVD (Adriamycin, Bleomycin, Vinblastine, and Dacarbazine) chemotherapy for six cycles.
2. **Radiotherapy**: After completing chemotherapy, the patient underwent involved-field radiation therapy to the affected lymph nodes.

Outcomes:

- The patient experienced typical chemotherapy side effects, including mild nausea and fatigue, which were managed with supportive care.
- Follow-up scans showed complete remission, with no evidence of disease after treatment completion.

Lessons Learned:

- Multimodal treatment for pediatric Hodgkin lymphoma is highly effective, with excellent cure rates when therapy is administered appropriately.
- Early identification and management of side effects are essential to maintain quality of life and treatment adherence in pediatric patients.

Case Study 4: Colorectal Cancer with Metastasis

Patient Profile:

- **Age**: 62
- **Gender**: Male
- **Diagnosis**: Stage IV Colorectal Cancer with Liver Metastasis

Treatment Plan: The patient presented with abdominal pain and weight loss. Imaging revealed primary colorectal cancer with multiple liver metastases. The treatment plan consisted of:

1. **Chemotherapy**: The patient was started on a regimen of FOLFOX (Folinic acid, Fluorouracil, and Oxaliplatin) combined with targeted therapy (bevacizumab).
2. **Surgical Intervention**: After four cycles of chemotherapy, the patient underwent a liver resection for the largest metastasis.
3. **Adjuvant Chemotherapy**: Following surgery, the patient continued on FOLFOX for additional six cycles.

Outcomes:

- The patient responded well to chemotherapy, with significant tumor reduction noted in imaging.
- Post-surgical pathology showed no residual cancer in the resected liver tissue, indicating effective treatment.

Lessons Learned:

- The combination of chemotherapy and targeted therapy played a crucial role in managing metastatic colorectal cancer.
- Coordination between medical oncologists and surgical teams ensured timely interventions, optimizing treatment outcomes.

Conclusion

These case studies illustrate the diverse treatment approaches in radiotherapy and chemotherapy across various cancer types. Each case highlights the importance of individualized treatment planning, the role of multidisciplinary teams, and the need for ongoing monitoring and support. By learning from real-world experiences, healthcare providers can enhance their practices, improve patient outcomes, and contribute to the advancement of cancer care.

In the final chapter, we will summarize the key insights from the book and discuss the future perspectives in cancer treatment, reflecting on the evolving landscape of oncology and the promise of ongoing research and innovation.

Chapter 25: Conclusion and Future Perspectives

Summarizing Key Insights and Envisioning the Future Landscape of Cancer Treatment

As we conclude our exploration of "Mastering Radiotherapy and Chemotherapy," it is essential to reflect on the critical insights gained throughout this book and to envision the future landscape of cancer treatment. The advancements in oncology have transformed how we approach cancer care, providing hope and improved outcomes for patients worldwide.

1. Key Insights

Multidisciplinary Approach: One of the most significant insights from this book is the value of a multidisciplinary approach to cancer treatment. Collaboration among oncologists, radiologists, nurses, dietitians, and mental health professionals is crucial for delivering comprehensive care that addresses the complex needs of cancer patients.

Personalization of Treatment: The move toward personalized medicine is a game-changer in oncology. By utilizing genomic profiling and biomarker testing, clinicians can tailor treatments to the individual characteristics of each patient's cancer. This approach enhances treatment efficacy and minimizes unnecessary side effects.

Advancements in Technology: Emerging technologies in radiotherapy, such as IMRT, SBRT, and novel chemotherapy agents, are revolutionizing how we treat cancer. These innovations allow for more precise targeting of tumors while sparing healthy tissue, leading to improved outcomes and reduced side effects.

Importance of Patient Education: Educating patients about their treatment options, potential side effects, and self-management strategies is critical for empowering them in their care journey. Informed patients are more likely to adhere to treatment regimens and report concerns promptly, leading to better management of complications.

Integrative Approaches: The integration of complementary therapies into cancer care is gaining recognition for its role in supporting patients' physical and emotional well-being. Mind-body techniques, nutritional support, and psychosocial care contribute to a holistic approach that enhances quality of life during treatment.

Focus on Safety and Quality Assurance: Maintaining safety protocols and quality assurance measures in both radiotherapy and chemotherapy is paramount. Continuous monitoring and adherence to best practices ensure patient safety, minimize risks, and optimize treatment efficacy.

2. Future Perspectives

Looking ahead, several trends and considerations will shape the future of cancer treatment:

1. Continued Innovation in Therapies: Research and development will continue to yield new treatment modalities, including more effective immunotherapies, targeted therapies, and personalized treatment strategies. Innovations in gene editing technologies, such as CRISPR, hold promise for potentially curative approaches.

2. Increased Use of Artificial Intelligence: The integration of AI in oncology will revolutionize diagnostics, treatment planning, and patient monitoring. AI algorithms can assist in identifying patterns in patient data, optimizing treatment strategies, and predicting treatment responses.

3. Emphasis on Survivorship Care: As cancer treatment improves, the focus on survivorship care will grow. Addressing the long-term effects of cancer treatment, including physical, emotional, and psychological challenges, will be vital for ensuring the well-being of cancer survivors.

4. Global Access to Cancer Care: Efforts to improve access to cancer care worldwide are essential. Addressing disparities in treatment availability, particularly in underserved populations, is crucial for ensuring equitable access to life-saving therapies.

5. Patient-Centered Care Models: The future of oncology will increasingly prioritize patient-centered care models that focus on the individual needs and preferences of patients. Engaging patients in their treatment decisions and providing comprehensive support will enhance the overall patient experience.

6. Collaborative Research Efforts: Collaborative research initiatives, both nationally and internationally, will be essential for advancing cancer treatment. Sharing data, resources, and expertise will foster innovation and accelerate the development of new therapies.

Conclusion

"Mastering Radiotherapy and Chemotherapy" has provided a comprehensive overview of the current state of cancer treatment, highlighting the importance of integrating various approaches to enhance patient care. As we look to the future, the combination of technological advancements, personalized medicine, and a commitment to holistic care will undoubtedly continue to transform the landscape of oncology. By fostering collaboration among healthcare providers and prioritizing patient-centered approaches, we can improve outcomes and quality of life for individuals affected by cancer.

In closing, the journey of mastering cancer care is ongoing, and the insights gained from this book serve as a foundation for future advancements. Together, we can continue to innovate, educate, and support patients in their fight against cancer, ensuring that they receive the best possible care on their path to recovery.

www.ingramcontent.com/pod-product-compliance
Lightning Source LLC
Chambersburg PA
CBHW082109220526
45472CB00009B/2107